A fitness plan for every woman who wants to look better, feel better and live her life more fully!

Based on the proven results, research and ongoing studies of the basic AEROBICS program, here is the first Aerobics book written especially for women! It will: tell you why today's women have a particular need for Aerobics exercise; explain the medical, physical, emotional and cosmetic benefits of the popular program; make specific suggestions for exercise during menstruation, pregnancy, menopause and other conditions; report on the personal Aerobics experiences of women across the country; offer a special chart-pack of exercise programs geared specifically to women of all ages and a brand-new point evaluation system for activities that most women engage in every day, as well as special high-priority health and beauty exercises.

AEROBICS FOR WOMEN
The modern way to keep fit and slender

aerobics
FOR WOMEN

**Mildred Cooper
and
Kenneth H. Cooper, M.D.**

BANTAM BOOKS
TORONTO · NEW YORK · LONDON · SYDNEY

ACKNOWLEDGMENT

Except for the contribution made by Nancy Spraker Schraffenberger in the preparation of this manuscript, AEROBICS FOR WOMEN would never have been possible. Both of us want to express our sincere appreciation.

AEROBICS FOR WOMEN

A Bantam Book / published by arrangement with M. Evans and Co., Inc.

PRINTING HISTORY

Evans edition published June 1972

Bantam edition / January 1973

2nd printing . February 1973	11th printing . February 1977
3rd printing . . . . . June 1973	12th printing . . . . . June 1977
4th printing . . January 1974	13th printing . December 1977
5th printing . . . . . June 1974	14th printing . . February 1978
6th printing . . . March 1975	15th printing . . . August 1978
7th printing . . . . July 1975	16th printing . . . . . April 1979
8th printing . December 1975	17th printing . November 1979
9th printing . . . March 1976	18th printing . . . . April 1980
10th printing . . . August 1976	19th printing . December 1980
	20th printing . . . April 1982

ISBN 0-553-22723-8

Published simultaneously in the United States and Canada

PRINTED IN THE UNITED STATES OF AMERICA

29 28 27 26 25 24 23 22 21

Contents

To women everywhere who have cared enough about their own physical well-being to undertake an aerobics program.

Dr. Cooper Regrets . . . and Rectifies

AFTER I WROTE my first book, *Aerobics,* and before my second, *The New Aerobics,* was published, I received a letter from Marie R. Gill of Potsdam, New York, from which I humbly quote:

> *I write this in an utter snit. I'm reading your book,* Aerobics, *and am convinced the program will mean a lot to me. I can hardly wait to start.*
>
> *But—at one point you say there are only two types of people, men and women, and that body differences, musculature, et cetera, are no excuse to earn less than 30 points.*
>
> *All right, you acknowledge us as part of the human race. Where do you deal with our problem? I find a short section, most uncomplimentarily tacked on the end of a chapter on special groups including such "odd cases" as Over 50 and The Fat Boys' Club. No wonder we are in such bad shape.*
>
> *How can we consider ourselves important when we're relegated to obscurity? You have no program for females—just a passing suggestion that we might aim for a 9-minute mile. Phooey!*

I have to admit that Mrs. Gill was by no means the only member of the fair sex to accuse me of unfair treatment. Well, I plead guilty with extenuating circumstances.

My first book was really designed for young Air Force men. But the response from outside the military was so enthusiastic, particularly from people past 35, 40 or 45 years of age, that we saw immediately we had to make some changes.

In the second book, age-adjusted scales were included for all the specific exercise programs, along with a lengthy chapter addressed exclusively to women's fitness needs, attitudes and capabilities.

And still the response from women was so strong in terms of eagerness, questions and correspondence about special problems that a book devoted—in fact, restricted—to their use was no longer merely an appropriate sequel to the first two; it was mandatory.

When *Aerobics for Women* became inevitable, the most natural thing in the world for me to do was to ask my wife Millie to collaborate with me in writing it. As I said in the dedication lines in *The New Aerobics,* Millie has been my tireless co-worker, my unwavering supporter—and she is a beautiful example of the benefits of consistent exercise. Besides the fact that she lectures regularly and authoritatively on aerobics to groups throughout the country, she has something that I cannot begin to approach with all my scientific investigations: a woman's understanding of women.

So, together we've prepared this new book based on continuing aerobics research, current fitness studies on women, case histories and a wealth of personal experience in talking and corresponding with American womanhood.

Thank you for your patience—and bless all of you who cared enough to complain.

KENNETH H. COOPER, M.D.

Dallas, Texas

What about Liberating Your *Body?*

LONG BEFORE KEN or I had the remotest idea that I was going to be Mrs. Cooper, a mutual friend asked him, "Would you like a date with Millie?"

"Not in a million years!" he said. "That girl never stops talking—she just yaks all the time."

How we got from there to here is another story. But one thing I've learned (apart from the value of listening): I can talk about aerobics till I'm blue in the face and it doesn't do a bit of good until *you* can say, "I *know*." You have to taste it and experience it yourself to know the exhilaration that comes from being in good physical condition.

Beauty is *not* skin-deep. There's a radiance and a glow in every woman who's active—in the way she carries herself, in the way she looks, feels and lives. A lot of women exist till 90, but they never *live* past 20.

In these pages, I'll be urging you—relentlessly—to live.

MILLIE COOPER

Dallas, Texas

1: One Woman's Liberation— From Fat, Fatigue and Apathy

I SIT HERE now, thinking about what aerobics has done for me in terms of my figure (dress size down to size 8 from size 12), my weight (down 10 to 12 pounds), my energy and sense of well-being, the luxury of eating what I please without worrying about calories and my freedom from tension and insomnia, and I feel rather smug.

But I also have to wonder how Ken must have felt 10 years ago when he was studying exercise physiology— knowing he intended to devote his life to this field, and knowing too that his wife couldn't care less about it. If he couldn't convince *me* of the health benefits and sheer pleasure that come from having a fit, conditioned body, how could he convince anyone else?

You may think you're indifferent to the subject of exercise, but you couldn't find anyone more tuned out than I was when Ken and I were married in 1959.

We're both natives of the Sooner State (we grew up 20 miles apart without crossing paths) and we also met in Oklahoma at the Fort Sill Army Base in Lawton. Ken had just finished his internship and was fulfilling his military obligation as a flight surgeon and I, fresh from the University of Oklahoma with a degree in sociology, had a job there as a recreation director with special services.

I come from a family that suffers from a disease common to 50,000,000 Americans: obesity. (Incredible as it seems, 25 percent of this country's population is at least 15 pounds overweight.) My sister used to tip the scales at over 200 and my grandmother died weighing close to 300 pounds. I never had a weight problem while I was growing up because I was active—I played girls' basketball and in college I took the required physical-education courses—but like many others my family certainly didn't encourage regular exercise as a way of life.

On the other hand, Ken's family had always been exercise-conscious. His father is a dentist who instilled in him a deep appreciation of the value of preventive medicine, and his mother encouraged him in athletics. During his high school years he was Oklahoma state champion in the mile (time, 4:31) and when I met him at Fort Sill, running and jogging were as much a part of his daily routine as brushing his teeth. I viewed his concern with fitness as a mild eccentricity (but it certainly wasn't a deterrent when he proposed).

In those days before joggers had become a familiar sight, people who saw you running in a public area thought you were being chased or going to a fire. I was always being asked, "Is your husband that nut who runs all the time?"

Truthfully, exercise to me was strictly for athletes and body-builders. I couldn't imagine anyone making a career of it. I used to wish Ken would go into pediatrics so I could say he was a baby doctor—everyone knows and respects *that* field.

Instead, he switched from the Army to the Air Force because of his interest in the aerospace program and eventually we were transferred to Boston so he could work on his master's in public health and doctorate in exercise physiology at Harvard.

If I nurtured any illusions about life in a big, conservative New England city influencing my husband against running in public, they were short-lived. I soon learned that I was up against the Boston Marathon. His determination to compete in this 26-mile foot race, staged every April for amateur runners, made him even more avid about his daily exercise. To train for it, he ran every day in every kind of weather, including −10° temperatures that actually froze his nostrils. Naturally, he'd wear his most beat-up old clothes, and most days he'd pass the same two newspaper boys doing their route. Once he heard one remark to the other, "Hey, look, here it comes again."

That pretty much expressed the way I felt when I'd see

him. After running 10 miles, he'd ride his bicycle 8 miles to Harvard. I'd drive our car to work and turn my head when I passed him. I found the whole thing acutely embarrassing. (When the Boston Marathon was run, he placed 101 among 400 competitors.)

You might well wonder what earthshaking event converted me from such negativism about exercise. It was the swift and steady beating of my own heart.

After Ken finished his course work at Harvard we were stationed at Brooks Air Force Base in San Antonio, where he began to specialize in research relating to the particular exercise needs of the astronauts. I still wasn't exercising regularly, although I'd occasionally go bike riding with Ken. Our daughter Berkley was born and then I was totally housebound for the first time. I had that after-pregnancy dumpiness and dragginess. One night Ken and I were relaxing after dinner, watching television, and he said, "Take my resting heart rate."

So I checked his pulse—and got about 50 beats a minute. Then he counted mine and got 80 beats.

"Thirty beats' difference isn't so much," I said blithely.

"Oh, no? Think of it this way," said my cagey husband. "While we're asleep tonight, your heart is going to beat about ten thousand times more than mine will. Even though our hearts are pumping the same *amount* of blood, it takes your heart that much more work and effort to do the job because you're not in condition. You're just going to wear out faster than I will."

Do I need to elaborate on what went through my head, including visions of Ken, a widower, courting the woman who would become the second Mrs. Cooper—and Berkley's stepmother?

The combination of these dire thoughts with the fact that deep down inside I secretly admitted that Ken was right about the need for daily exercise and the benefits of it, finally persuaded me that I couldn't afford *not* to get into an aerobics conditioning program.

The next day I put Berkley in her stroller, hitched our

dog on her leash and started pushing and pulling all of us over a mile-and-a-half course that Ken measured out for me around our neighborhood in San Antonio.

An exercise program *has* to be individual if it's to be successful. Fortunately, aerobics offers plenty of options: you can walk, jog, run, skip rope, climb stairs, swim, bicycle—do any number of activities or sports that stimulate your heart and lungs over a prolonged period of time. Several of the options weren't feasible for me because of Berkley or because they just didn't appeal. (I don't enjoy water sports. As a result, Ken and I have never shared one of his favorite recreations, water skiing, and I have an almost worshipful admiration for any woman who earns her aerobic points by swimming.)

I decided to make running "my thing" because it was handiest and I could take Berkley with me. At that time it was convenient for me to run in the late afternoon and that was when I seemed to need it most. I got through the day fine, but about four o'clock I'd find myself getting headachy, irritable and lethargic from being cooped up in the house.

The first few weeks were the very hardest because I was just starting and knew I couldn't expect results right away. It was like a diet, I'd think, "I just can't do this." But somehow each day I'd manage to put on my track shoes and get me, my child and my dog on the road again. First I'd walk, and then I got to the point where on downhill sections I'd start jogging—it must have been quite a spectacle, me pushing Berkley in her stroller with her red hair standing up on end, and a fat blond cocker lumbering along behind.

On Sundays, Ken and I would run together. He'd put Berkley in the stroller and let me get to the top of the hill in front of our house and then they'd start out behind me. Little Berkley would yell "Faster, faster, Daddy," and I'd hear them gaining on me even though I had a half-mile start. I felt insulted that they could catch me, so I started trying harder on my daily workouts during the week. In time, the effort paid off in far more than being able to outdistance my husband and daughter.

I became two sizes smaller. I've always been heavy

through the hips and I took off 4″ in that area alone. My dress size went from 12 to 8.

I weighed less. You don't lose a lot of weight rapidly from exercising, but you do convert fat to lean muscle and you lose inches. This, combined with the fact that the exercise curbed my indulgent appetite, resulted in a weight loss of over 10 pounds. Of course, a reduced-calorie diet *with* exercise is marvelous; you burn up 100 percent fat. (If you fast without exercise, you burn about 50 percent fat and 50 percent muscle mass.)

My eating habits were automatically controlled. Although you may not lose weight on an exercise program by itself, you definitely won't gain. I love to eat, and what a pleasure to enjoy a dessert or between-meal snack and know I wasn't going to pay for it in pounds because I was burning them up!

At the same time, I found my desire for rich goodies was not as keen. When I came back from exercising, the thought of a piece of cream pie was nauseating, but sucking on a fresh orange was just great. Also, people who exercise regularly crave more fluids, and drinking a lot of fluid is a good way to control appetite.

I was less tense, more energetic and slept better. Exercise banished my end-of-the-day blahs. I built up a second wind and felt less tired in general. And I had no residual tension to keep me awake when I went to bed.

My resting heart rate decreased from 82 to 57 beats per minute. My entire heart/lungs/blood-vessel system became more efficient. This was evident not just from my lower heart rate; I actually breathed easier. Lungs are like balloons and most of us breathe out of the top half only. Getting air down into the lower half isn't easy at the beginning—it's like trying to inflate a new balloon for the first time. But after you're conditioned, you feel a real difference in the ease of air flow in and out.

My self-image was definitely enhanced. Even if you *couldn't* document everything that happens to a person physiologically as a result of aerobics, which you can, the psychological benefits are worth everything. I know I don't lose a pound or an inch every time I run, but I know how good I feel when I do something to improve myself and my figure. In one area of my life, at least, I have discipline. No matter what else happens during the day, I can say to myself, "Well, I got my exercise in."

I was aware of my husband's pride in me. Before I started exercising, I'd watch a woman come up to Ken and say, "Dr. Cooper, I'm running a mile in such-and-such a time." The admiration that would come into his eyes really made me jealous. Now I can hear the pride in his voice when he tells other people what *I've* accomplished in my aerobics program.

As I said before, exercise is individual, as individual as the makeup you choose for yourself. It's got to fit your needs, your desires, what you're best at—walking, swimming, cycling, whatever.

Once you get into it, you're hooked: the smaller dress sizes, the good feeling about your body, your husband's pride, even the way other people envy your self-discipline.

Eventually, when Berkley started nursery school, I switched my exercise program to mornings so I could do it while she was being taken care of. Even then, after some conditioning, I never dreamed I'd ever be able to run a mile nonstop. It wasn't even my goal. I'd start off jogging, then walk a while, then jog a while. And every day I'd jog to the same point before I got tired.

One day I was jogging along, planning what to have for dinner, and when I looked up I'd *passed* the point where I always stopped before—yet I was still running and I was not fatigued.

Now this is the aerobic training effect. One day it's just there. What you couldn't accomplish the day before suddenly becomes a snap.

So every day I set *little* goals for myself—getting beyond a certain house, and so on. And every day I *inched* my way to running a mile nonstop, and it was the greatest feeling in the world to know I could do it. It's a fact that most people —men included—can't run a mile. If you happen to mention that you *can*, people look at you and marvel. Being able to excel at something unusual does wonders for your self-esteem.

For example, one day I went out to the air force base where Ken was testing some young WAF's of 18 or 19. He was running them on a mile test and said, "Why don't you run with them?"

I was 32 or 33 then, at least 10 years older than those girls, and it was a challenge. I started running with them and after the first quarter-mile, scads of them began to poop out—in fact, my 16-year-old niece ran with us and she finished last. I came in second. Can you imagine what it felt like to know, at my age, I was in better shape than those dewy young recruits?

Shortly afterward, a man-woman running event was held at the base—the woman would run the first mile, then pass the baton on to the man and he'd run the next 2 miles. Ken and I won first place in our age category. Another triumph that meant more than merely winning!

DON'T TAKE MY WORD FOR IT

When you consider that the United States Air Force has adopted aerobics as its official fitness program, it must be clear that I haven't been brainwashed and that my experience is far from unique. But from the standpoint of personal testimonials, I wish we had space to quote from every one of the thousands and thousands of conversations we've had and the letters we've received from women all over the country telling us of their individual results with the program. For now, I'll content myself with just one comment, unsolicited, from Mrs. Pat Neumann of Bloomington, Indiana, describing the aftermath of her 12-months' aerobics running program:

> One year ago my figure was apparently a phenomenon. In a store, a salesclerk called over another to demonstrate the amazing fact that I was a size 12 at the waist, yet a size 20 nine inches lower down. (She didn't make a sale.) I don't know how long it was that each thigh measured bigger around than my waist. You've never seen a more vastus lateralis, nor a gluteus more maximus.

Now all that's changed. One day last spring I was leaning over making a bed and happened to notice one of my knees. In alarm, I wondered what awful bony growth I'd developed, so I quickly checked out the other knee. The same. I finally realized I was looking at my knees themselves, revealed from under the blobs of fat they'd been hidden in for years. I've never been overweight, but when about 90 percent of any excess is deposited exactly, literally, in one quarter of your height, the effect is that much more grotesque.

I've found that every one of my measurements has improved through running, whether the need was for a decrease or an increase. I fill a bra for the very first time in my life, and the other part of me I'm glad to see built up is my calves. When a gal's lower legs are too close to being all one circumference at ankle and calf, it sure is pleasing to read a tape measure at a new lower number for the ankles and a higher number for the calves. But lest my talk of buildup frighten off someone who doesn't need or want it, let me emphasize that the change is from ugly, lumpy-pillow flab to nice lean muscle.

I'd like to emphasize, too, that measurements are only a small aspect of the picture. The spontaneous reaction of men and women acquaintances who hesitate, step back and exclaim, "Hey, you look good! What've you been doing?" makes a very happy me. Much more important is the reaction of my husband, whose appreciation flows on and on. Which brings us to a problem of yours, Dr. Cooper. How are you ever going to write in a book that from aerobic exercise a husband will enjoy far more improvement in his wife than just her new appearance? After all, there are other senses besides sight!

2: You're Already an Aerobe, What More Do *You* Want?

AT THIS POINT, you're probably wondering exactly what aerobics is. First let me give you a 5-year-old's version.

We've never talked specifically about "aerobics" to Berkley, but it certainly is a well-worn word around our house, and little children are powerfully observant. One day she said to me, "Where's Daddy?"

"He's out talking to some people," I answered. "Do you know what he's talking about?"

" 'robics."

"What *is* aerobics?" I asked, trying not to show how curious I was about her ideas.

"Running, swimming, riding a bike."

"Why does somebody want to do those things?"

"Makes you healthy. Makes you feel good."

Those answers are absolutely correct, as far as they go. It's not true, however—as Berkley and probably a lot of other people think—that Ken made up the word "aerobics." It's pronounced *a-ró'-biks* and you'll find it in Webster, defined as "living, active or occurring only in the presence of oxygen."

Women or men, we're all aerobes, meaning we need the presence of air in order to survive. Ken stretches the term "aerobics" when he uses it in connection with exercise to mean "promoting the supply and use of oxygen."

Here's how it translates: Activity of any kind demands energy. Your body gets this energy by burning the food you eat. Oxygen is the igniting factor and the food is fuel. Your body can store up food, but it's not able to stockpile oxygen.

From the meals you eat—3 a day are ample for most people—the body spends whatever is necessary for current

19

energy needs and "banks" some of the remainder in the form of fat tissue. You can go for a reasonably long time without eating and still survive. But with the igniting agent oxygen, the body's demand equals the supply, and the supply has to be maintained on a minute-to-minute basis by breathing. Without breathing, the oxygen present in the body would be rapidly depleted and every vital organ would quit. To be blunt, you would die.

All this, admittedly, is common knowledge. But Ken's point is that some of us breathe better than others. Some of us breathe efficiently enough to get a rich supply of oxygen to every nook and cranny of the body where food is stored and to produce energy in abundance. Others just don't get enough of it around fast enough. They are the easily tired ones who can't seem to keep going, the physically unfit as opposed to the aerobically fit.

As an example, suppose a group of us were called upon for a quick action requiring sustained effort—say we were picnicking together and looked up to see a child some distance away in danger of falling into deep water. Suppose we all jumped up and started running as fast as we could. This is what would happen to the body as it strained forward: The chest would heave as the lungs sought more oxygen, the heart would pound as it strove to push more blood through the body (blood transports the oxygen) and the blood would race in its effort to deliver more oxygen to every remote part.

Shortly after we started to run, some of us would start to fall back. But those who were conditioned would get there first because they could take in oxygen faster and use it more efficiently. Or to put it another way, the people who were not aerobically conditioned would run out of energy quicker and reach the exhaustion point sooner. They simply could not process oxygen as well as the others.

The classic argument is, "But I don't *need* that much energy on a day-to-day basis. How often am I called on to save an endangered child? Who needs that kind of endurance anyway?" We all do.

Chances are you're more than a little familiar with some

of the typical signs of a deconditioned body—being breathless after even small efforts like carrying grocery bags, mopping the floor, pushing the stroller a few blocks or running upstairs to answer the phone; yawning early in the day; nodding off at your desk; feeling too bushed to do much more than flop down in front of the television set at night.

These are the symptoms of inactivity and over a period of time the cumulative effect can be seriously damaging. If you don't use your body, it breaks down. Your lungs lose their efficiency, your heart becomes weaker and more vulnerable, your blood vessels tend to lose their suppleness, your muscles get flabby. The entire oxygen-delivery system is crippled.

AEROBICS FOR YOUR HEART, LUNGS AND BLOOD VESSELS

A few years ago, when we were living in San Antonio, I often took Berkley to the city zoo. One day, as we were passing the mountain goats' cage, we noticed that the animals—normally among the world's nimblest—had trouble with their footing. A closer look showed us that their hooves had grown so big and shapeless that the poor goats were barely able to hobble around. In captivity, away from the natural environment where climbing over rough, rocky, hilly ground had kept their hooves in good, trimmed-down condition, they'd lost all their agility and freedom to caper and run.

The goats illustrate a short, succinct phrase Ken and I have for referring to the capacity of the heart: Use it or lose it. Everything from minds to muscles (and the heart is a muscle) atrophies from lack of use. During the past several decades, mechanical power has been replacing muscle power. This is just as true, if not more so, for the woman at home or in the office as it is for the man on the job. We've put motors on everything—typewriters, sweepers, pencil sharpeners, mixers, even toothbrushes. As recently as the time when our grandmothers were young, women got substantially more exercise during a routine day than they do in 1972.

I know what you're saying to yourself at this point. I've heard it before. When I lecture I invariably meet more than one woman who says, "Don't tell *me* I don't get enough exercise, Mrs. Cooper. Every day all day long I do housework, do for the kids, wash, iron, cook. . . ." And I know that many women who work outside the home will claim they're not exactly sedentary in their jobs, either.

Two misconceptions are lurking here. So let's set them straight. One: feeling tired doesn't necessarily mean your body has been adequately exercised. The tired feeling more often than not represents mental fatigue from the pressure and tedium of having to get so many routine things done during the day. Real physical exercise actually erases mental fatigue. By the time you've cooled down from aerobic exercise, you're practically recovered from the physical exertion and you're beginning to feel refreshed and relaxed in mind *and* body. That's why so many ulcer patients exercise at the end of the day, when they're emotionally keyed up and mentally fatigued. With exercise, they seem to neutralize the acid that's poured into the stomach.

Second, no matter how vigorously you've wielded your mop or paced around your office, you haven't done a thing for your heart-lungs-circulatory system. What you've done is exercise your muscles. This kind of activity concentrates on only one system of the body, one of the least important ones. It has a limited effect on your essential organs and allover health. What you need is the kind of exercise that will demand oxygen and force your body to process and deliver it. And that's what aerobics does.

Exactly what kind of physiological changes can you expect from aerobics?

- You'll breathe easier because the muscles in your chest wall will be stronger; air can flow in and out more rapidly and with less effort. When you do tiring work, your body will take in more oxygen to produce energy.
- You'll distribute oxygen more rapidly from your lungs to your heart to all parts of your body because your heart will beat more strongly and pump more blood

with each stroke. This reduces the number of strokes necessary. Even when you're working hardest, your heart will pump blood at a lower rate than if it were deconditioned.

- You'll increase the number and size of the blood vessels that transport blood to your body tissue, thus enriching tissue all over with more oxygen for energy.
- You'll have more blood circulating in your body—more red-blood cells and more hemoglobin to carry the oxygen.
- You'll tone up all the muscles and blood vessels in your body and enjoy better blood circulation in general; a frequent additional side effect is lowered blood pressure.

These exercise-induced changes in the various systems and organs of the body are known collectively as the *training effect* of aerobics.

AEROBICS FOR YOUR HEALTH AND WELFARE

To help you decide whether aerobic exercise has any application to you personally from the physiological standpoint, here's a group of ten yes-no questions.

	Yes	No
1. My physician is satisfied with my weight.	——	——
2. I have adequate control over my eating, smoking and drinking habits.	——	——
3. I can run a few blocks or climb a few flights of stairs without becoming short of breath.	——	——
4. My resting heart rate is usually in the efficient 55-to-70 beats per minute range. (As a test, sit and relax for five minutes, then check your pulse for a minute against a watch or clock with a second hand.)	——	——
5. My doctor says my blood pressure is normal.	——	——
6. My heredity gives me nothing to worry		

about in terms of heart or lung disease
or diabetes. —— ——

7. My blood vessels seem to be healthy
enough—for example, I don't have a problem with varicose veins. —— ——

8. I rarely have trouble with acid stomach,
heartburn, indigestion and the like. —— ——

9. I'm seldom if ever constipated. —— ——

10. I have nice firm muscle tone—no flabs
or sags. —— ——

If your answer to any one of the above questions is "no,"
you ought to think seriously about an aerobics exercise
program.

What is an aerobic exercise program? Simply put, it's
doing a certain amount of specific exercise 4 or 5 times a
week—walking, jogging, running, swimming, cycling, any
number of familiar activities—long enough to push your
heart rate up to 130 to 150 beats a minute, depending on
your age and the duration of the activity. (Of course, no
one but a conditioned person can do that without first
building up to it on a graduated exercise program, and that's
the purpose of Ken's age-adjusted, week-by-week charts.)

I've suggested one set of motives for getting into aerobic
exercise—the physiological. Now let me offer some psychological ones.

AEROBICS FOR YOUR EGO

Your reason for exercising doesn't matter in the least.
I freely admit that my heart and lungs are abstractions to
me (and I think they are to most people). But I no longer
take their good work for granted. People will never rave
about "how well my heart and lungs are looking"—that's
a private and profound gratification, just for me. But they
do rave about other things, and the tangible, visible, pride-
giving results of my aerobics program are what keep me
persevering.

On the psychological, ego-building side, here are ten
questions to help you discover what *your* reasons might be:

	Yes	No
1. I'm satisfied with my weight, my body's contours and the dress size I wear.	——	——
2. I get sincere compliments on my appearance from my family and friends.	——	——
3. I'm proud of my accomplishments—and so is my family.	——	——
4. I feel I'm just as attractive as the other women in my group.	——	——
5. I eat what I please and don't worry about calories.	——	——
6. I can get through the average day without feeling tired and depleted.	——	——
7. I feel fit and energetic and eager to start each day.	——	——
8. I'm seldom tense, irritable, or depressed.	——	——
9. I sleep beautifully and wake up feeling refreshed.	——	——
10. I feel confident that I'm doing my best for my body, inside and out.	——	——

If you checked "no" for even one of these questions, you've got a good reason for going aerobic.

As I said before, my own reasons are a combination of physiological and psychological. Over the long haul, I want to do everything I can to prolong my life with my husband and children—our son Tyler arrived in December 1970—and to make my body healthy enough to enjoy that life to the fullest. On a day-to-day basis, I love knowing my figure is at its most attractive, I love being able to wear clothes in the most flattering styles and sizes, I love the compliments from my husband and friends.

AEROBIC EXERCISE FOR YOU, A WOMAN

To go back to the beginning, all human beings are aerobes. But pathetically few of us are aerobically fit, even though it's common knowledge that heart and blood-vessel disease kills more people in this country than war or traffic accidents or all other diseases combined.

No matter how many aerobic benefits can be documented and cataloged, Ken feels that only one aspect of this exercise program is crucially important and that is its potential contribution in changing the statistics on death and disability from heart disease for men and women. He *can't* guarantee that aerobics will prevent a heart attack or enable you to live even one day longer. But he does insist that "grooming" your cardiovascular-pulmonary system is the best single hedge against heart disease and that it will put life into the years you do live and make them more productive and enjoyable.

However, as a result of the lab and field tests he has conducted on thousands and thousands of subjects, Ken has also come to the conclusion that women don't need to develop quite the same level of fitness that men do in order to have the same protection and pleasure. In short, they can progress more slowly to a level that's different from —but equal to—the one men achieve. Let's look at the differences between men and women more closely.

3: You Are Not a Man

PROBABLY YOU'VE HEARD the saying that goes something like, "Every fat man is a prison for a thin man yearning to be free." Certainly most men care about looking good and keeping their weight down. However, we've observed that these things are usually lower down on their totem pole of priorities. A man gets seriously interested in aerobics not from the standpoint of his physique but because he has a friend who just 10 days ago died of a heart attack. He knows he's more susceptible to heart disease than a woman and he thinks of living longer, seeing his children grow up —and like many people in this country, he may have made a lot of money and wants to be around to enjoy it.

American males lead the world in deaths from heart disease, and the most alarming increases in cardiac conditions are among men in their thirties, forties and fifties.

On the other hand, we women—up to an age that varies individually with the onset of menopause—have the advantage of a kind of built-in immunizing factor provided by the female hormone estrogen. During our childbearing years, we have traditionally ranked behind men in death from heart disease because our bodies produce this hormone.

Estrogen is, in fact, such a significant factor in reducing coronary disease in women that at one time physicians actually experimented with injecting it into men, particularly after they'd already had a heart attack. Unfortunately, so much estrogen was required to achieve protection that it also produced a feminizing effect. The men started developing breasts, losing their beards, experiencing voice-change —this therapy proved impractical, to say the least.

At this point I'd better hasten to say that having estrogen is no reason for smugness. When you go into menopause, the production level of this hormone declines and there's

27

a corresponding rapid increase in the frequency of coronary disease among women. Moreover, as Ken puts it, the time has passed when women can sit back complacently and rest on their hormones.

With the new laws against discrimination by sex and the new thinking about placing women in high-level executive positions, more and more of us are accepting the same strenuous or stressful jobs that have literally taken the heart out of American men. Ken suspects that handling more of this job pressure and male-type stress reduces the protective effect of estrogen. And for *all* women, stress from any source—combined with other factors such as obesity or weight gain, inactivity, high blood pressure or cigarette smoking—can diminish the hormone asset.

The point is, aerobic exercise is more essential in the age of women's liberation than ever before.

MALE VS. FEMALE

Estrogen accounts for a major chemical difference between men and women. As for physical structure, girls mature earlier than boys until puberty, the age at which we first become capable of sexual reproduction, varying from 12 to 14 or so. During puberty, boys develop their longer, heavier bones, additional body weight and greater muscle mass. Girls, meantime, are acquiring the fat deposits that provide the soft, rounded contours associated with femininity (and sex appeal). These fat deposits also give us a special aptitude for floating in water. Another noticeable structural difference between women and men is, generally, our wider hips and the slightly different angle in the way the head of the femur—thighbone—is set into the hip socket, giving our walk a circular motion compared to the more straight-forward action of a man's stride. Obviously this affects our manner of running and our capacity for it.

Ken's own studies and information from other researchers indicate that boys reach their maximum natural fitness—top aerobic capacity for heart output and lung intake—in their late teens and early twenties. For girls, the peak comes during puberty to the middle teens. From these ages on, the fitness level for both sexes declines unless they maintain it with exercise.

Fortunately, society is beginning to change its very rigid ideas about what constitutes appropriate "feminine" and "masculine" behavior. Many stereotyped notions seem to be in decline, and a woman can excel in a sport or be vigorous and dedicated in her approach to exercise without also being the subject of ridicule and raised eyebrows.

In addition, increasing numbers of people are becoming aware that those old myths about exercise causing a woman to develop bulbous muscles and an unappealing, unfeminine physique simply aren't true. It's just the other way around —and I'm not too modest to point to myself as one of several million living, breathing examples of the opposite effect. Another specific example, one much admired by Ken, is Elaine Peterson, a United Airlines stewardess and stewardess instructor who's also an accomplished marathon runner. She competes in 4 or 5 long-distance events every year, including the Boston Marathon, and you've never seen a better figure or lovelier legs—or at least Ken says *he* hasn't!

EXCLUSIVELY FEMALE

So far, I've been fairly general about the physical differences between men and women. But what about the parts and processes that are exclusively female? Starting from the top, you can imagine how many women have asked about the effect of exercise on breasts, and whether bust size will tend to increase, decrease or remain the same.

As in so many instances, it's impossible for Ken to make an unqualified statement. We get a substantial number of letters from women who say they've noticed an increase or decrease in size, and in almost all cases the change—in either direction—has been considered a desirable one by the writer.

We do know for certain that exercise tends to firm up all body tissue, including that of the breast, and that flexion, contraction and extension activities with the arms—the kind that go with swimming or swinging your arms as you run— can build up the pectoral muscles supporting the breasts.

Ken's recommendation to all women, particularly those with large bosoms, is that they wear a firmly supportive bra when they exercise. This is not only more comfortable, but it also helps protect the ligaments supporting the breast, which are anatomically known as the ligaments of Cooper (no relation).

As for tearing of tissues, abscess formation or tumor development, exercise doesn't have any connection with these breast problems.

Next, the menstrual cycle. Here's an area where most doctors agree: reasonable physical exercise during menstruation is not just allowed, it's often helpful, especially to women who experience dysmenorrhea—painful menstrual periods. Any exercise that improves blood circulation and muscular strength and flexibility in your abdominal region is desirable and frequently relieves the discomforts of cramps and lower-back ache, as well as the logy feeling. A conditioned body is simply better prepared to handle this monthly stress. As a matter of fact, world records have been approached by Olympic stars performing during their menstrual periods!

Granted, some women have such a heavy first-day flow that exercise on that day is just impractical, and granted also that incapacitating monthly pain surely calls for treatment by a physician—but otherwise I urge you to discover that exercise can be beneficial to you whether your periods are normal or nerve-racking.

AEROBICS AND MATERNITY

This subject has to be discussed in three parts: before pregnancy (in relation to those women who want to have babies, but aren't getting anywhere), during and after.

Again, no promises are implied, but we have some examples where exercise appeared to have a positive influence on fertility. These were cases of women who seemed to have sterility problems, yet became pregnant after starting an exercise program. One explanation, Ken believes, is that chronic fatigue—which can affect the normal menstrual cycle—may also be disrupting to the ovulatory pattern. Exercise dissipates habitual nervous fatigue, the tensions and stress that can cause these irregularities, and may help re-establish a normal pattern.

To cite a personal example, we have friends in Oklahoma who adopted, over a period of time, three children after several years of trying to have a baby on their own. Just about the time they adopted the third child they both started on an exercise routine and within twelve months the wife was pregnant.

Since they had a history of adoptions, the psychological aspect of commitment to a baby wasn't involved, as it is with many couples who adopt their first child and then achieve pregnancy. The only new factor for this pair was exercise and Ken feels, as they do, that exercise played a significant role.

The wife enjoyed a wonderful freedom from pregnancy problems and discomfort, too, which brings up the question of exercise during the gestation period.

This letter from Mrs. Byron Bowles of Lee's Summit, Missouri, is a typical one from our large "P for Pregnancy" file.

> When my husband and I started the aerobics stationary-running program in mid-July, I was three months pregnant. My doctor was very much in favor of exercise so long as I built up slowly and switched to something less strenuous, like walking, during the last few weeks. This I did.
>
> We had had three children before this one, so I had a basis for comparison. I'd also been active in the past and consequently had thought I was in pretty good shape but I was certainly fooled.
>
> This pregnancy was unbelievably easy and recovery was extremely rapid (I started running again when the baby was 2 weeks old). Also, the baby came when due

instead of early as the others did. He was heavier by more than a pound.

I can't think of a better time in a woman's life for her to have the benefits of this program. Good circulation is really vital for an expectant mother. Exercise and pregnancy would seem to be a good subject for a study by obstetricians.

The twenties and thirties are the most active childbearing years, and it's obvious that if a woman wants to have a strong body during the time she is reproducing—the period when she's having to carry the extra weight—she needs to build up tissue and muscle tone. We all know that among native women in remote tribes it's not at all uncommon for an expectant mother to give birth in the morning and then go ahead with her daily activities without slowing down for a minute. These women are so much stronger—their tissues and muscles are so much healthier—that they can more easily tolerate the stress of pregnancy.

There's no question that if you build up the supporting muscles of your stomach, particularly the abdominal muscles, labor will be facilitated. The other important area in which exercise is helpful is in strengthening the back. (Back pains are one of the chief complaints during and after pregnancy because a woman's center of gravity has moved down about a foot and a half and she has to walk around with a curvature of the back to support her abdomen.) And the list goes on: exercise can help in reducing the swellings and the abnormal collection of fluids that may come with pregnancy; with constipation; with leg cramps.

The problem of varicosity bears special mention. Varicose veins occur when a muscle loses its tone and a vein its elasticity; blood tends to pool there, causing a dark, ugly spot. These discolored veins appear in 10 percent of all pregnancies (more often in women who are already excessively overweight) and Ken believes that by building up the muscles and veins through exercise, varicosities can be avoided, reduced and sometimes eliminated.

In short, exercise is definitely a bonus to pregnant women

who aren't experiencing complications such as constant abdominal pain or vaginal bleeding, and moderate forms of outdoor activity are wholeheartedly recommended. Explicitly, Ken says: "First, consult your obstetrician. If he feels exercise is permissible, I would allow even jogging up to the sixth month. After that time, I would suggest milder forms of exercise such as walking, stationary cycling or swimming. (Although some women have continued to jog almost until delivery with excellent results, this decision should rest with your obstetrician.) When exercise can be resumed after delivery is a debated subject. Intuitively, I'd suggest waiting about 6 weeks, even though I have records, like Mrs. Bowles', of women who've started as early as 2 weeks after childbirth. In any case, *do* anticipate taking up your exercise program again. Your reward, among other things, will be the return of your youthful figure."

Few women are exempt from after-the-baby blues. In my experience, one cause of postpartum depression is feeling so misshapen and not being able to get into my slim, trim "normal" clothes, and I can attest that aerobics helps. Six weeks after having our little son Tyler, I'd lost only 20 pounds of my birth gain. I wasn't exercising and I couldn't diet because I was breast-feeding (nursing helps prevent your gaining weight, but it didn't help me lose). I started jogging again and lost 6 pounds in 3 weeks *without* dieting.

Exercise after pregnancy is your ally in helping firm up muscle and tissue tone and in deflating the traditional "beach-ball belly." And it's immensely valuable in dispelling the backaches that often persist after you've had a baby.

AEROBICS AND MENOPAUSE

Now, making a seven-league stride from childbearing to nonchildbearing years, let's talk about menopause, the last of the exclusively female processes. I doubt that it will surprise you if I make a strong case for aerobic exercise at this time of life. In fact, I consider it a must.

Foremost, there's the diminishing-estrogen factor discussed

at the beginning of this chapter. Second, as a woman gets older, she's more subject to elective-type surgical procedures, and whether they involve gall bladder or stomach operations or removal of a breast, her chances of having postoperative complications are much reduced if she has kept herself physically fit.

In connection with breast surgery, I want you to hear the story of one of the most remarkable women we know, Myrtle Pehrson of Excelsior, Minnesota. Mrs. Pehrson is 52 years old, five times a mother and twice a grandmother. In her words:

I joined the YWCA in 1954 for the exercise and swimming programs and 4 years ago I started jogging.

In March 1970, the doctor discovered I had cancer of the breast and at the end of the month a radical mastectomy was performed on my left side. Because of my good condition, no skin graft was required to mend the incision and I responded so well to therapy that they didn't have to use a breathing machine on me. The doctors couldn't believe how well I could move and help myself. Instead of being in intensive care for 4 or 5 days as expected, I was out in 48 hours.

Five days after my surgery I was informed that the other breast would have to be removed in 7 or 8 weeks. I went home and did the exercises the hospital gave me, plus any others I felt able to do. I was ready for the second surgery at the end of April, exactly 4 weeks after the first.

By the first of June I was swimming and by July I was playing 18 holes of golf. In September I went back to the Y and in no time I was back to jogging 3 or 4 miles a day 3 times a week.

The doctors had me on a special diet because my cholesterol count had gone up to 330. I weighed 105 pounds at the time. I didn't stay on the diet, but after two months of jogging my cholesterol count was down to 211.

Whether it's a matter of preparing yourself for procedures like this or of assuring yourself of a longer life by lessening the possibility of coronary disease, the older woman who is conditioned and has good muscle tone will face fewer problems. She's going to be able to keep her youthful-looking tissues, her youthful-looking legs, her youthful-looking skin. (Ken has a woman patient of 73 who's an avid walker and, without exaggerating in the slightest, he compares her legs to Marlene Dietrich's.)

Finally, Ken believes that some of the changes characteristic of menopause—hot flashes, hormone imbalances—may be attenuated to some extent by regular exercise. He also predicts, while admitting that he can't substantiate the statement, that the psychological trauma of menopause will be reduced if a woman has maintained a fit body.

AEROBICS FOR WOMEN—THE DIFFERENCE

To sum up, both sexes benefit from aerobics, absolutely, though for men to exercise or not to exercise may be even more of a life-or-death decision than it is for women.

None of the uniquely female processes by themselves prohibit regular, hearty exercise; rather, these functions make it a desirable option and often an urgent need.

The aerobics programs in Ken's first two books have been implemented successfully throughout the world—they've been translated into several languages—but these programs were not designed for women.

Aerobics for men includes taking a 12-minute walking/running test to discover the individual's fitness level, and earning 30 aerobics points a week. (The aerobic point system, which enables you to measure your progress and work toward an appropriate fitness level by degrees, is fully explained at the beginning of the next chapter.)

Neither of these requirements applies to women.

In recent years, as his research has progressed, Ken has determined that most women's total aerobic capacity is smaller than most men's, in keeping with our generally smaller physical size. Our hearts are usually smaller physically, as is our lung capacity; we have less blood circulating and thus less hemoglobin and fewer red-blood cells.

Consequently, he no longer feels it's necessary for a woman to achieve the 30-points-a-week goal he specifies as the requirement for a man to reach a good fitness level. On the basis of continuing studies, he has found that in working up to 24 points a week a woman can reach a satisfactory level of fitness. (Naturally he doesn't discourage women who choose to exceed that goal and are physically able to do so.)

Moreover, he sees no need for a woman to take a fitness test unless she especially wants to. Simply by achieving 24 points' worth of aerobic exercise a week she can be assured that she's physically fit.

In a nutshell—aerobics for women is equal, but easier.

For quick reference, here are the new aspects of aerobics for women and where you'll find them described in this book.

• *Optional* aerobics fitness test based on running, plus 3 new optional fitness tests using swimming, cycling or walking, Chapter 6, pages 52-54.

• Progressive, age-adjusted (under 30, 30-39, 40-49, 50-59, over 60) aerobics exercise programs for women based on running, walking, rope skipping, stair climbing, swimming, outdoor and stationary cycling, Chapter 8, pages 64-82.

• Caloric value of about a hundred common foods and beverages with amount of aerobic exercise required to prevent weight gain, Appendix, pages 156-159.

• Exercise selector for burning up specific caloric amounts, Appendix, page 160.

• Combination exercise "menus" for the housewife with a park nearby; for the woman who wants a well-rounded program and owns a stationary bicycle; for the tennis player who owns a bicycle; for the jogger with tennis and golf skills; for the dating girl, Appendix, page 155.

• New point evaluations for favorite forms of dancing, for walking while pushing a carriage or stroller with a baby in it, for sports and recreation activities popular with women, Appendix, page 154.

4: If Your Heart's Not in It, It Isn't Aerobics

IF I HAVEN'T made it abundantly clear already, I feel bound to emphasize that you can't earn aerobic points with a passive, pitty-pat effort that leaves you looking as if you'd just stepped from a bandbox. Obviously, if you're going to burn enough oxygen to make your heart beat in the 130-to-150-beats-per-minute range I mentioned earlier, you've got to work your body pretty hard.

Notice that I said "work *your* body." That phrase explains Ken's answer to the enthusiastic horsewoman who asked him how much aerobic credit she got for riding an hour every day. "*You* don't get any credit," he had to tell her. "It all goes to the horse."

THE AEROBIC POINT SYSTEM

In the lab and field tests Ken conducted with thousands of Air Force personnel as well as civilians, he was able to establish a correlation between certain levels of oxygen consumption and popular forms of exercise. Each exercise requires a certain amount of energy and therefore a certain amount of oxygen. Ken measured the amount of oxygen it "cost" the body to perform various exercises and translated the various amounts into aerobic points. The more energy expended in a certain time, the more points you get; the less energy, the fewer points.

For example, in the aerobics running program, walking a mile in 15 minutes is worth 1 point; running 2 miles in 25 minutes is worth 4 points.

For all women, Ken has established that the *minimum* number of points necessary to produce and maintain a satisfactory level of fitness is 24 per week. Older women simply work up to this level more slowly. All any woman needs to reach this goal are the point, distance and time charts in Chapter 8, a watch with a sweep second hand and the will to persevere. (You may be wondering about the 130-150 heartbeat range—how are you supposed to count your heart rate while you're exercising? No problem—it too has been figured into the point system.)

PROGRESSIVE LEVELS

Since it would be dangerous for you to try to build up from a stage of doing no exercise to the 24-point level of aerobic fitness too quickly, Ken has broken the various exercise programs into 10- to 18-week stepping-stones, the number depending on your age category. To return to the example of jogging or running, a woman under 30 would progress from walking a mile in 17 minutes 5 times a week during her first week to earn 5 points . . . to running a mile and a half in 13½ minutes 4 times a week for 24 points by the end of the tenth week. On the other hand, a woman between 40 and 49 would progress from walking a mile in 19 minutes 5 times a week to earn 5 points at the beginning . . . to jogging a mile and a half in under 14½ minutes 4 times a week to earn 24 points by the end of the fourteenth week. The 4-week difference in the length of the program reconciles the difference in age.

Don't let the number of weeks suggested in the exercise programs become a magic figure. Some people may take twice as long to reach the 24-point level. The amount of time doesn't matter, only that you work up to the 24 points eventually. If you find it too difficult to make the goal for any given week, you simply stay at that level and work toward that particular week's goal until you can *comfortably* achieve it.

I do want to emphasize that you can get the aerobic training effect in two ways: over a long period of time with the low-intensity effort that walking calls for; or over a short period of time with a high-intensity effort of the kind jogging or running requires. Either way is satisfactory.

After you've completed the aerobics exercise program of your choice, you don't have to limit yourself to one form of conditioning. You can combine whatever exercises you wish to earn your 24 points weekly (see the suggestions in the Appendix, page 155).

When you're just starting, though, stick with *one* aerobic exercise and go through the complete program. It's not advisable to switch from one to another until you've completed a full program—your muscles become adjusted to a certain type of exercise and you may not be able to keep up your rate of progress if you take on a different form before you're fully conditioned.

You can exercise 4 or 5 days in a row or every other day. But Ken feels it's better *not* to exercise 7 days a week because of chronic fatigue. You do need time off to rest.

One important thing to remember after you've reached the 24-point level is *not* to try to earn all your points in one day, then skip exercising for the next 6. You've got to earn your points over a spread of least 4 days. You can earn 5 points one day, 1 point the next, 9 the next, and so on, as long as they add up to 24. In between days of formal exercise, you can pick up points just by walking.

AEROBIC VS. NON-AEROBIC EXERCISE

Ken's measurements of points, distances and times relate only to aerobic exercise—cardiovascular-pulmonary conditioning. But as you well know, there are many other forms of exercise. What are the differences between them and aerobics?

Exercise can be used in three different ways. In one, it's used as a means of rest and relaxation—the sheer enjoyment you get from a few holes of golf or playing with the kids. It's fine to get as much of this as you can, but don't count it as cardiovascular conditioning. In the second group, exercise is used for figure contouring and muscle building. Much can be said in favor of building up beautiful figures in women and firm, muscular bodies in men, but if you do this to the exclusion of aerobic exercise you'll never be truly fit. Finally, exercise can be used to build up cardiovascular and pulmonary reserves. The three are not interrelated. The first two can be valuable, but doing either one—or both—does not give you the benefit of the third.

Exercise for figure control and muscle building—the second group—takes in some "brand names" you're probably familiar with. I'd like to explain fully what they are, and why they aren't aerobic.

Isometrics This involves contracting a muscle without moving a joint. Pulling the knob of a locked door is an example. Isometric exercises enjoyed a great vogue in this country in the 1950's and 60's, a vogue that hasn't quite died out because they are billed as a shortcut: sweatless exercises accomplished in a minute or two a day. Unfortunately, their effect is also to shortchange you. Isometrics work is done only on muscles around bones—no benefit whatever to your heart, lungs or blood vessels. If you want to become a champion puller-on-locked-doors, and not much else, confine your exercise program to isometrics.

Isotonics Here a muscle is contracted to produce a range of movements. Examples are calisthenics, weight lifting, bowling. More dynamics are involved than in isometric exercise, but still it's mostly the skeletal muscles you're conditioning, not the cardiovascular-pulmonary system. The trouble is that calisthenics don't demand enough oxygen, or if they do the demand doesn't last long enough to be of any benefit.

That much said, let me quickly add, before I lose all the women who swear by calisthenics, that both Ken and I appreciate this form of exercise and use it ourselves as a *supplement* to aerobics. I like to warm up with calisthenics before I start my daily jog—I'll describe the ones I do later—but in no way can they be considered a substitute for aerobics.

Anaerobics. Now we're getting close to aerobics, but not close enough. Anaerobics make your body demand large amounts of oxygen, but not for a sufficient period to be of real value to your heart and lungs. Remember the example I gave of running a distance to rescue a child? That would give you anaerobic exercise. So would active, stop-and-start sports like gymnastics, and athletic events like the hundred-yard dash. But, like your vacation, they don't last long enough.

Aerobics differs from recreation, isometrics, isotonics and anaerobics in that you pick an activity and gradually—over a period of several weeks—build your body up to demanding large amounts of oxygen for a sustained length of time.

THE AEROBICS CHOICE

Whatever your circumstances—wife, mother, career woman or all three—and whether you live in the city, suburbs or wide-open spaces; whether home is a house, trailer or apartment, aerobic exercise can be adapted to your life-style. Not only is it as free as the air you breathe, but it's varied enough to—well, to nullify every excuse you might think up for *not* doing it.

Confined to the house? Do an indoor exercise like stationary running, stair climbing or rope skipping. Work from nine to five? Walk part or all of the way to or from your office. Get babies to keep an eye on? Take 'em along. One mother we know of straps her 35-pound toddler on the extra seat over the rear wheel of her bicycle. Don't like that sweaty feeling when you exercise? Swim. Hate to go it alone? Jog with a friend. Prefer privacy? Mrs. Robert Showalter of Martinsville, Virginia, created her own, exclusive indoor track:

In our basement we have a large family room on one side and three smaller rooms on the other, and I noticed that if all the doors were open in all four rooms you could run through all the rooms without having to stop. We measured the exact distance we would be running in one lap with string and determined that it would take 76 laps to make a mile. So there was my running track—not the most ideal, for sure, but it does have the advantages of both privacy and a place for the baby.

I find running exhilarating. And I was amazed at the immediate improvement in my physical condition. Every afternoon when my 9-year-old son comes home from school we run a mile. Then after dinner he runs another mile with his Daddy (who started regular exercise after he lost a bet with us that he could run a mile in 10 minutes). We're enjoying every minute!

AGE CODING WITH EXERCISE RECOMMENDATIONS

Whether you're 70 or 17, your age isn't a barrier to aerobic exercise. You'll simply work toward the 24-point level at a different rate, using Ken's age-adjusted standards. He has established 5 different age brackets:

Under 30
30 — 39
40 — 49
50 — 59
Over 60

The chief difference in using the exercise charts if you're over 30 is that you'll move to the desired fitness level more slowly.

Ken also has guidelines for what form of aerobic exercise is sensible and safe according to your age.

Under 30: Free choice, unless you have a medical problem of some sort.

30-49: Free choice, but get your doctor's permission if your inclination is toward the more vigorous exercises.

50-59: Condition yourself with a walking program before you contemplate anything more strenuous, and have a medical checkup before embarking on something like jogging or running.

Over 60: Walking, swimming and stationary cycling are encouraged, unless exercise has been a well-established habit. Let your past experience and your physician's advice be your guide.

MEDICAL CHECKUP

No matter what your age is, it's mandatory that you have medical supervision in connection with your exercise program.

Under 30: If you've had a medical checkup in the past year and received a clean bill of health, you can start any time.

30-39: The medical history and physical examination should have taken place within the past six months.

40-49: The history and examination should have taken place in the past three months and should have included an electrocardiogram (ECG) taken while resting.

Over 50: Same as 40-49, except the examination should be given immediately before starting into an exercise program and also should include an ECG while exercising. Your pulse rate should reach the level expected during strenuous aerobic exercise.

On the subject of age, I'd just like to add that I participated in a 40-mile "Miles for Children" walking/running marathon to benefit the March of Dimes in San Antonio in 1969, and I never could have gone the distance if I hadn't been inspired by my constant companion on the trek: a woman in her seventies.

5: A Cautionary Tale for Contemporary Women

SINCE PAGE 1, I've been giving you autobiographical anecdotes and clinical information on the benefits of aerobics from the standpoint of self-esteem and, most importantly, as preventive medicine. For the most part, I've been talking about my own experience and that of other "average" women who enjoy lives relatively free from sickness or even menacing symptoms of sickness—women who have never had a real scare in terms of their health and well-being.

But present membership in this privileged group carries no lifetime guarantees. Like the men in this country, American women are also world champions in those depressing statistics on death by heart disease. Just one example: the current figure on coronary fatalities among French women between ages 35 and 44 is 3.5 per 100,000 population each year. In the United States, for the same age bracket and population unit, it's 18.5. That's a tremendous 5-1 ratio in our "favor."

To me, even grim numbers like those are too remote and anonymous to be deeply meaningful. I find my own moments of truth in individual cases. Can you imagine the physical and emotional effects of a heart attack on a young woman with a young family? It happened to Mrs. Jeffrey Paxton (she prefers that we not use her real name), who has become one of Ken's patients, and her story is enough to make *any* woman pause and reflect.

The Paxtons have three children. They're very well off financially, meaning their income provides a big, beautifully furnished home, unlimited travel, all the creature comforts. Mrs. Paxton is now 42, an attractive, slim, small-boned brunette. Until the time of her coronary "ambush," she was energetic and active. But when Ken first saw her she was a cardiac cripple and a cardio-neurotic—literally terrified of making the slightest move for fear of endangering her heart, utterly panic-stricken under her passivity.

This is Mrs. Paxton's account in her own words, taken from my notes.

"I've never been described as a relaxed person. For one thing, I'm a nonsleeper—a nocturnal animal. When the house gets nice and quiet I'd rather read than go to bed. I've been a two-packs-a-day smoker since college. I'm definitely not the calm type.

"Both my parents are living, but they both have heart disease. At age twenty-one, I developed a problem known as a 'rapid heart'—it's *not* a form of heart disease, but it scares the devil out of you. The comparison would be to racing a car motor. The acceleration can last anywhere from ten minutes to all day long. I'd have it once every year or two —very unhandy, but you get used to it.

"I never got exercise on a daily basis before my attack. My husband had read Dr. Cooper's books, and at one point he tried to get me interested in conditioning. I said, 'Ha! At the rate I move, if you tried to follow me around the house all day long you'd be exhausted. *You're* the one who needs exercise, not I.' Me, the world's authority.

"At the time of my attack, I had no weight problem, no warning symptoms, never had had surgery, and I wasn't menopausal either. But the other factors—heavy smoking, hypertension, no exercise, my parents' history—were evidently enough to do the trick.

"It happened in July 1970, during what was supposed to be a pleasant little family vacation. My youngest child and I were going to pick up my son Teddy at a camp in New Mexico and then go on to visit Canyon de Chelly and the Grand Canyon. My husband couldn't join us, but he helped us map out the trip and planned so we wouldn't have to drive too far each day.

"By the time we left Las Vegas, New Mexico, after collecting Teddy, I had a funny sensation in my chest, as if I needed to belch, but I figured it was the unaccustomed seven-thousand-foot altitude. Anyway, we drove on. The kids were excited and so was I—we were having such a good time.

"At Canyon de Chelly we took the morning tour and when we got back I definitely felt strange. I analyzed it, in my supreme ignorance, as too much heat, so I skipped lunch, except for tea and eating a little salt, and felt better. Before we headed on to Grand Canyon it did occur to me to get myself checked by a doctor in Gallup, but I let the thought pass.

"We took the northern route up the side of the canyon, a winding road that seemed like the end of the world— dramatically beautiful and completely desolate. I thought we'd never get there. I was uncomfortable every mile of the way and started taking Tums for my 'indigestion.' After dinner that night, I felt better again and we went to bed early. The next morning we did some sight-seeing. I didn't feel great, but not too bad. But driving away from the canyon my hands started to shake and I pulled off the road. I knew I was awfully close to fainting.

"I told the kids to flag down a car because I wasn't feeling well, and an Army captain stopped to help us. My last gesture before entering Grand Canyon Hospital was to light up a cigarette. Smoking didn't cross my mind again for quite some time because I was put in an oxygen tent and hospitalized there for the next three and a half weeks.

"At Grand Canyon my condition wasn't diagnosed as a heart attack, so my shock-reaction was somewhat delayed. They said it was cardiac insufficiency. But when I returned home, my local doctor, an internist, called it a myocardial infarction, the first time that term had been used.

"I don't know which was more devastating, realizing that I had had an attack, or going into our beautiful bedroom at home for the first time and seeing that an enormous oxygen tank had been installed. I had a fit. 'What in blazes is this doing here?' I said to my husband.

" 'Doctor's orders,' and I wound up taking twenty or thirty minutes of oxygen after every meal, griping all the way.

"Normally, I have anything but a lethargic disposition, but I didn't seem to perk back up after the attack. My doctor told me, 'Look, you didn't get this way overnight, you're not going to recover overnight. It might take three or four years.' How frustrating! You think, 'Okay, if that's the way it's going to be . . .,' yet something in you protests.

"Anyway, I made up my mind that if I must, I had enough discipline, control and skill to handle my life from my bedroom.

"Basically, the prescription was bed rest. And my constant complaint *was* tiredness. I just couldn't seem to get my strength back. I also suffered the fear of not knowing how much to try. You don't want to harm yourself, yet you're so anxious to get going again. Another complication—I developed a skin rash, which was treated with cortisone. I reacted to it with chest pain, which frightened me horribly.

"In December following the attack I contacted Dr. Cooper and made an appointment with him. Not surprisingly, he found me very tense.

"First of all, he gave me a history form to fill out, we chatted for a while, he took my blood pressure and so on. Over a period of time, he did a blood work-up, and I had ear and eye examinations (arterial damage can show up in the eye).

"On this first visit, he put electrodes on my chest and did what he calls a resting cardiogram, measuring my heart rate as I rested. And then he put me on a treadmill! I thought, 'I can't run—what are they trying to do, kill me?'

"Actually, as I learned, this is not an unusual procedure. The electrodes remain fastened to your body to give exact recordings of your heartbeat pattern as you walk or run. In other words, you're monitored by very sensitive equipment the entire time. My performance was pathetic—in less than three minutes I'd had it.

"Part of what they were determining was whether I *could* exercise. Some people who've had bad heart attacks can't vigorously exercise ever again. Of course, this was my great apprehension, that my worst fears about being disabled for life would be confirmed.

"They weren't. The verdict: 'Very slowly we'll start to exercise you on the treadmill here in the office.' It *was* slow, too. We went from five minutes to ten minutes over a period of weeks, and gradually the treadmill speed was increased. But by the seventh week, I went a mile in sixteen minutes, compared to my first-day snail's pace, which was equal to going a mile and a half in an *hour*.

"At the beginning I did all my exercise in Dr. Cooper's office. I wasn't allowed to do anything at home, and nothing alone. This restriction continued for a month. Now I exercise five times a week unsupervised—on a treadmill at home or with fast walks, just under a jog, with my husband.

"When I started the exercise program, I did minimal house chores except for getting breakfast. I had a cook in the evenings. Today I no longer have the cook. Even on the phone, people tell me, 'You don't *sound* the same.' I guess there's more energy in my voice, too. Well, I feel good, better than before the attack. I don't think I'll ever be completely without tension, but I do seem able to cope more easily now. I'm much more relaxed because I'm not as frightened—it's that simple. These days I'm getting six to seven hours of sleep a night and I also rest in the afternoons.

"If you're able to achieve discipline in one area of your life, it seems to carry over into other things as well. You get pride in handling yourself. It's pretty disgusting to be forty-two years old and *know* you shouldn't smoke, for example. I knew I had enough problems already without adding cigarettes to them, yet if I hadn't succeeded in incorporating the exercise routine into my life, I'm certain I would have gone back to smoking.

"Maybe while I was pulling my heart and my leg muscles out of atrophy, I was also reactivating my brain. Obviously, during the time I was 'calming' myself with cigarettes and 'curing' myself with rest, I was also deteriorating.

"I think it should be stressed that women are changing their living patterns. Because of the way we're directing our lives, the future, for us, is not unlike that of the male. We'll reap what we sow."

6: On Clothes, Climate and Your Own Physical Condition

MY FOND HOPE is that you're willing, eager and able to start your aerobic conditioning this very minute, but there are a few more aspects of aerobics to fill you in on—some questions that invariably come up—before we get to the charts for the actual exercise programs.

Certain medical conditions absolutely prohibit your undertaking any form of an exercise program. These are:

- Moderate to severe coronary heart disease that causes chest pain (angina pectoris) with minimal activity.
- Recent heart attack. A 3-month waiting period is mandatory before you start on a regular conditioning program, and even then any conditioning must be medically supervised.
- Severe disease of the heart valves, primarily the result of having rheumatic fever at an early age. Some patients with this condition shouldn't exercise at all, not even to the extent of walking fast.
- Certain types of congenital heart disease, particularly those in which the body's surface turns blue during exercise.
- Greatly enlarged heart resulting from high blood pressure or other types of progressive heart disease.
- Severe heartbeat irregularities calling for medication or frequent medical attention.
- Uncontrolled sugar diabetes constantly fluctuating between too much and not enough blood sugar.
- High blood pressure not controlled by medication— for example, readings of 180/110 even with medication.
- Obesity. If you're more than 35 pounds overweight according to standard charts, you must lose weight on a walking program before you can begin anything more strenuous like jogging or running.

- Any infectious disease during its acute stage.

In addition to the 10 restrictive conditions listed above, Ken has designated another group of 10 ailments that don't forbid exercise, but they do make caution and a doctor's supervision imperative. As a matter of fact, exercise—the kind and quantity to be determined by your personal physician—may be beneficial to the health problems that follow.

- Any infectious disease in its convalescent or chronic stage.
- Sugar diabetes controlled by insulin.
- Internal bleeding, recently or in the past (in some cases, exercise is not permitted at all).
- Kidney disease, either chronic or acute.
- Anemia under treatment but not yet corrected (less than 10 grams of hemoglobin).
- Lung disease, acute or chronic, that causes breathing difficulty even with light exercise.
- High blood pressure that can be reduced only to 150/90 with medication.
- Blood vessel disease of the legs that produces pain with walking.
- Arthritis in the back, legs, feet or ankles, requiring frequent medication to relieve pain.
- Convulsive disease not completely controlled with medication.

KNOW YOUR CAPACITY

The first rule of aerobics is: Never get ahead of yourself —or of the charts. Rushing just doesn't work and only invites trouble. Work up to your goal gradually. This is important not only to accustom the heart to the new demands, but also to let tendons and muscles adjust themselves to the new activity. Once you and your doctor have decided there's nothing to prevent your starting the exercise program of your choice, you can use certain simple guidelines to tell whether you're pacing yourself properly as you go along.

Personal Stress Gauge Indications that you're overdoing

your exercise are: a feeling of tightness or pain in your chest, severe breathlessness, light-headedness, dizziness, losing control of your muscles, nausea. If any one of these symptoms crops up, it's a clear signal to stop exercising immediately.

Your Heart-rate Response To find out if you're exercising too hard for a woman in your condition, check your "recovery heart rate." Five minutes after exercising, take your own pulse. (If you can't find your wrist pulse strongly enough for an accurate count, put your palm over your throat and check it there.) Use a watch with a sweep second hand and count the pulse for 10 seconds, then multiply by 6. Or count for 15 seconds and multiply by 4.

If the count is over 120, you know you're overextending yourself. Ten minutes after exercising, check your pulse again. Now it should be down below 100. If not, it's a sign to cut back a bit on your exercise.

Your Breathing-rate Response If you're still short of breath 10 minutes after exercising, that's a further indication of overexertion. As a comparison, the normal breathing rate at rest ranges from 12 to 16 breaths a minute.

OPTIONAL FITNESS TESTS FOR WOMEN

The fact that 4 fitness tests are included here doesn't mean that Ken is reneging on his statement that women don't have to take them. Rather, he wants the option of taking one to be available. We're aware that many women will be curious to know exactly where they place in the previously established aerobic fitness categories (I-Very Poor; II-Poor; III-Fair; IV-Good; V-Excellent). The tests are offered only to provide the means of pinpointing the level of physical conditioning.

If you're under 30, have had a medical examination within the past year and have no medical problems, you have the *option* of taking any one of the tests at any time. If you place in Categories IV or V, you can then feel free to start earning your 24 (or more) aerobic points without going through a basic program. If you place below Category IV, assign yourself to the appropriate age category in the exercise program of your choice and follow it through.

If you're over 30, DON'T take any fitness test until you've observed the medical precautions specified on page 43 *and* completed one of the basic programs. This done, you have the *option* of taking a fitness test to determine the level of conditioning you've reached. If it should be below Category IV, resume your aerobic conditioning program and slowly work up to 35-40 points a week using the expanded point systems in the Appendix. However, remember that 24 points per week is consistent with a good level of fitness, regardless of the category reached on one of the fitness tests.

The running test involves running and walking as far as you can *comfortably* in 12 minutes. You run until you're winded, then slow down until you get your breath back, then run again. However, since it's a test of your maximum capacity, it's important to push yourself as much as you reasonably can.

You can ascertain the distance you cover in two ways. Make use of an existing measured track at your local high school or YM/WCA—or mark off your own track in the park or on a low-traffic road using your car's odometer as a guide. You'll need a watch with a sweep second hand to calculate your time accurately—and it's a big help to have someone with you to do the timing. No special preparation is necessary for your run other than a few limbering-up calisthenics (trunk circling, toe touching and others on pages 61-62). Dress comfortably and pick a time when you feel rested and relaxed.

WOMEN'S OPTIONAL 12-MINUTE RUNNING TEST
Distance (Miles) Walked and Run in 12 Minutes

FITNESS CATEGORY	Under 30	30–39	40–49	50–59	60+
I. Very Poor	< .95	< .85	< .75	< .65	Not Recommended
II. Poor	.95–1.14	.85–1.04	.75– .94	.65– .84	
III. Fair	1.15–1.34	1.05–1.24	.95–1.14	.85–1.04	
IV. Good	1.35–1.64	1.25–1.54	1.15–1.44	1.05–1.34	
V. Excellent	1.65+	1.55+	1.45+	1.35+	

< means "less than."

The swimming test calls for swimming as far as you can in 12 minutes, using whatever stroke you prefer and resting as you need to, but basically trying for a maximum effort. The easiest way is to do it in a pool whose dimensions you know, and again, it helps to have someone along to record your laps and to monitor the time with a watch with a sweep second hand.

WOMEN'S OPTIONAL 12-MINUTE SWIMMING TEST
Distance (Yards) Swum in 12 Minutes

FITNESS CATEGORY	*Under 30*	*30–39*	*40–49*	*50–59*	*60+*
		AGE (years)			
I. Very Poor	< 300	< 250	< 200	< 150	< 150
II. Poor	300–399	250–349	200–299	150–249	150–199
III. Fair	400–499	350–449	300–399	250–349	200–299
IV. Good	500–599	450–549	400–499	350–449	300–399
V. Excellent	600+	550+	500+	450+	400+

< means "less than."

The cycling test, pedaling as far as you can in 12 minutes, can be done anywhere that you're likely to avoid being hung up by traffic—or getting an unbalanced amount of uphill or downhill terrain. The bike should be 3-speed or less and if it has an odometer you won't have to measure off the distance by other means (such as driving it in a car).

WOMEN'S OPTIONAL 12-MINUTE CYCLING TEST
(3-Speed or Less)
Distance (Miles) Cycled in 12 Minutes

FITNESS CATEGORY	*Under 30*	*30–39*	*40–49*	*50–59*	*60+*
		AGE (years)			
I. Very Poor	< 1.5	< 1.25	< 1.0	< 0.75	< 0.75
II. Poor	1.5–2.49	1.25–2.24	1.0–1.99	0.75–1.49	0.75–1.24
III. Fair	2.5–3.49	2.25–3.24	2.0–2.99	1.50–2.49	1.25–1.99
IV. Good	3.5–4.49	3.25–4.24	3.0–3.99	2.50–3.49	2.0–2.99
V. Excellent	4.50+	4.25+	4.0+	3.5+	3.0+

< means "less than."

The walking test, covering 3 miles in the fastest time possible without running, can be done on a track or over any measured distance. As with running, take the test when you feel rested and dress to be comfortable.

WOMEN'S OPTIONAL 3-MILE WALKING TEST (No RUNNING!)
Time (Minutes) Required to Walk 3 Miles

FITNESS CATEGORY	AGE (years)				
	Under 30	30–39	40–49	50–59	60+
I. Very Poor	48:00+	51:00+	54:00+	57:00+	63:00+
II. Poor	48:00–44:01	51:00–46:31	54:00–49:01	57:00–52:01	63:00–57:01
III. Fair	44:00–40:31	46:30–42:01	49:00–44:01	52:00–47:01	57:00–51:01
IV. Good	40:30–36:00	42:00–37:30	44:00–39:00	47:00–42:00	51:00–45:00
V. Excellent	< 36:00	< 37:30	< 39:00	< 42:00	< 45:00

< means "less than."

HEIGHT—YOUR OWN AND YOUR LOCALITY'S

Two special circumstances are questioned fairly often in connection with aerobic exercise. Mrs. Violet Bates of Loma Linda, California, brought up one: "Three of us have started the aerobics walking program. However, doesn't height make a difference? One woman is barely 5 feet tall, on is 5'2" and one is 5'10". The tall gal can cover a mile in 12 minutes with no more apparent difficulty than the shorter ones have in 14 or 15 minutes. Have you found that the length of stride has some bearing?"

Ken's answer is "yes." But it's interesting that height affects performance *only* in a walking program. Shorter women experience no disadvantage in running, rope skipping, stair climbing, cycling, swimming and so on. Here is Ken's adjustment for petite walkers: Comparing 2 women in the same age and fitness categories, the one less than 5'2" would earn 2 points for covering a mile in 16 minutes, while the one over 5'2" would have to earn her 2 points for the same mile in 14½ minutes. On all the charts for walking programs, women under 5'2" can give themselves this 1½-minute allowance on time goals.

Another "height" factor that deserves consideration is the altitude at which you're doing your exercise. It's true that the majority of people don't live in quite so rarefied an atmosphere as Mrs. Quentin Nordyke and her husband, American missionaries who serve in Juli, Peru, on the edge of Lake Titicaca—13,000 feet in the clouds. But the Nordykes and many others have asked Ken about the difference altitude makes in using the time goals. Adjustments are allowed for the extra effort expended when you walk or run in the thinner air at 5,000-foot altitudes and above. As a sample, 30 seconds are added to the time goals for jogging a mile at 5,000 feet; 60 seconds at 8,000 feet; 90 seconds at 12,000 feet. For a detailed chart on high-altitude exercise and compensations to make on the 12-minute test, see page 155 in the Appendix.

WEATHER OR NOT

I learned early in our marriage that the weather outside, miserable or not, won't deter my husband from running though his nose freezes over. But he's really quite scientific about what constitutes desirable conditions for other people who exercise outdoors.

Leaving out, for the time being only, the possibilities for exercising inside on a stationary bicycle or a treadmill, of stair climbing, rope skipping and stationary running—as well as running on indoor tracks and swimming in indoor pools —what about above-average heat and cold?

Let's start with the ideal: classic Cooper exercise weather is 40° to 85°F., humidity less than 60 percent and wind velocity under 15 miles an hour. Now back to reality.

The cardinal and common-sense rule is, don't overdo— don't exercise till you're exhausted, especially if you're just beginning a conditioning program. In summertime weather or tropical/semitropical climates, plan to exercise in the relative cool of early-morning or twilight hours. Remember to replace what you lose in perspiration by drinking lots of liquids, and do dress—I should say undress—for comfort. That means light, loose, nonconstricting clothing, anything regarded as decent in your neighborhood. Ken's cutoff points: no strenuous exercise when the mercury tops 95°F., particularly when the humidity is above 80 percent.

If you're exercising in cold weather, especially if it's accompanied by chilling winds, you should take some extra precautions in the way you dress. Don't make the mistake of putting on too many clothes or you'll perspire excessively

—wear just enough to keep warm. A surprising amount of heat is lost from your head area, so wear a pull-over-your-ears cap or a scarf or use the hood on your parka. Depending on your own sensitivity and the severity of the conditions, wear a knitted face mask as skiers do, or at least tie a muffler loosely over your nose and mouth to trap warm air. If you're perspiring freely after exercise, let yourself cool down gradually to avoid getting a chill.

Generally speaking, cold weather (even below-zero) holds fewer perils for exercisers than hot and shouldn't be a deterrent if you take normal precautions.

Unfortunately, another weather condition has achieved national prominence in recent years and must be given its due because considerable numbers of our population are affected. Mrs. Adryan Charnow of Los Angeles is one of many who've written to ask about it. "My husband and I chose the aerobic running program. Part of the area we run in is unavoidably a heavy traffic area, and what has bothered us about that is the smog. Our city has quite a problem, and even though we run in the early morning, I feel that breathing in all that soot and dirt could in some ways be harmful. Have you any information on this?"

Ken's reply: "To my knowledge, no harm comes from exercising in smog conditions—and I know of no studies documenting that smog has a detrimental effect on performance—even though it may tend to cause some irritation of the lungs and coughing. I think that to exercise and breathe in the smog is certainly better than to sit around and let your body deteriorate because you are afraid to exercise in it."

FASHIONS FOR AEROBICS

It's no exaggeration to use the term "fashion" in connection with clothing for exercise. Today, every sport from sailing to snowmobiling seems to have been supplied with its own wardrobe, and aerobics is no exception. The jogging and sweat suits being designed—coordinated two-piece outfits consisting of jackets or pullovers and pants with side zippers on the lower legs—are just as style-conscious and colorful as skiers' fashions.

"Dressing the part" may be good for your self-image when you exercise, but it isn't necessary to buy anything just for this purpose. More than likely, your closets and drawers are full of suitable clothing. Personally, I don't dress to look good when I run. Exercise time is not my most glamorous time of day—it's my personal time, like going to the beauty salon. I know I'm not my loveliest when I'm sitting under the dryer with my hair done up in rollers, but I know that the eventual result will be a prettier appearance.

For me, anything big and loose is fine when I exercise. I put on a big shirt and loose Bermuda shorts and when I get back from running I feel so skinny—those pants are just hanging on me.

The single item of apparel worth a special investment is shoes for walking, jogging and running (stationary or not). Your footwear can be a key factor in avoiding ankle, foot and leg problems. In walking a mile, for example, you subject the 26 bones in each foot to the full impact of your body weight at least 2,000 times. That's punishment!

The important built-in elements to look for in a running shoe are arch support, resilient insoles, rippled soles and a soft heel to cushion the Achilles tendon. Sporting-goods stores can guide you in your choice. Socks are a matter of personal option. I don't wear them, Ken does. Cotton ones are best for absorbing perspiration; nylon is not as absorbent but offers better insulation against friction.

To sum up the pointers on exercise clothing, any garment that restricts your movements won't be comfortable and may interfere with your breathing. Avoid tight bras and waistbands and never wear girdles, corsets or circular garters.

As for wigs, extra eyelashes and other "gay deceivers," you're on your own!

7: Before You're Off and Running (or Bike Riding, Rope Skipping, Etc.)

Now THAT YOU'VE seen your doctor and checked the weather and your wardrobe, are you ready for aerobics? Almost, but not quite. When you step into a conditioning program, it can be one of the most important steps you ever take and I want to make sure it's as fail-safe for you as humanly possible.

Assuming that you've established your own set of reasons for making exercise part of your life, prepare yourself to enjoy it—and to persist in it. I'd be the last person to claim that introducing a new habit into your daily routine and making it stick is easy. It isn't. As in dieting, the distance between your present state and the payoff can seem insuperable. Here are some gambits that may help you "psych" yourself.

Enlist boosters I can understand women who don't have much willpower because I'm one of them. I need continual bolstering (never hard to get when you're married to a Ken Cooper). Talking about your exercise program—sharing it —definitely helps. Tell your family and friends what you've set out to accomplish. Once they're interested, they'll encourage you—even if their boosting is in the form of teasing!

Try the buddy system Many women find their key to commitment in exercising in pairs or with a club. I know of an informal neighborhood group who like to run together after they get their kids off to school and before they face the demands of the day. These women say they enjoy postponing breakfast dishes and unmade beds in favor of their exercise because the workout inspires them to tackle the chores.

Think thrifty Aerobics doesn't take a single penny out of your purse. Imagine how much hospital costs would be reduced if more people practiced this sort of preventive medicine. For me, just seeing the bill for one day's stay in the hospital is enough to motivate me to get out and exercise.

Reward yourself Anyone who's dieted knows about the games you play to keep going—saving up calories from one day's ration in order to spend them on a big gourmet bash the next day, and so forth. I play similar tricks with my exercise. I tell myself, "If you run today, you can have some extra cookies with your coffee this afternoon." Take it from someone who lives to eat, I *do* want those extra cookies, but I won't have them unless I earn them. I refuse to pay myself for work I don't do.

Be realistic Don't make the mistake of setting an impossible goal for yourself. You're not expected to turn in an Esther Williams-Wilma Rudolph performance—just 20 or 30 minutes a day of exercise. Ken has carefully calculated all the aerobics exercise programs for reasonable, comfortable progress so that you're not inclined to overextend yourself to the point of discouragement. Don't dwell on the time goals or distances quoted at the end of the conditioning programs. Take your exercise on a day-by-day basis. In a remarkably short time, you'll discover, as I did, that you actually miss it if you have to skip a day.

Whatever form of mental winding up you do, follow it by deciding, once and for all, what time of day will be best for you to schedule your exercise and keep that time sacrosanct. Exercising at the same time each day is another way of reinforcing your commitment.

CHOOSING A TIME

Please yourself in picking a time of day to exercise. Just bear in mind that you shouldn't get involved in strenuous activity for at least 2 hours after eating a meal. For women who find that doing their stint first thing in the morning is a good eye-opener, and who don't want to exercise on an empty stomach, Ken suggests a glass of orange juice to "take the edge off" and provide quick energy. Wait 10 or 15 minutes after drinking it to start your exercise.

If you're not an up-with-the-larks type, midmorning or before-lunch exercise may suit you best. Moreover, vigorous preprandial exercise decreases your appetite. I keep comparing exercise with weight-loss programs because they're so much alike in the way you have to discipline yourself and establish a pattern. It's a natural thing to lose pounds while you're losing inches. Many people who exercise at noontime, for example, find it very easy to skip lunch, or they're content with a vitamin-fortified diet drink.

You'll experience the same tendency to eat lightly if you exercise before dinner, and I've already mentioned the soothing effect of late-afternoon exercise for ulcer patients or anyone high-strung.

Exercise close to bedtime may leave you overstimulated when you turn out the light—or you may be asleep before your head hits the pillow. If the former is true, change your timing to allow an hour or so of relaxation between exercise and sleep.

Being Faithful

One thing I tell women all the time when I'm a guest speaker at meetings: You can't store up physical fitness; there simply isn't a "layaway plan." Exercise is something you have to make up your mind to do daily or every other day.

Stop-and-start conditioning has no value whatever in building up your aerobic capacity. In fact, it can be harmful. Turning a light switch on and off does more to deplete the bulb's lasting power than letting it burn; on-again, off-again exercise is also an unsatisfactory way to prolong endurance.

To put it bluntly, be faithful to your conditioning program or leave it alone. I've trotted out all the excuses and none are valid for not finding the time to exercise except sickness, immunization (24-hour layoff period), all-out fatigue, extremes of temperature or weather (outdoor exercisers only!) and blessed events.

If you *are* called out of town or get sick or for some other reason have to interrupt your exercise program for more than a few days, make an allowance for the time lost. A certain amount of slippage will have occurred in your aerobic capacity—how much varies from person to person, but the older you are, the bigger the slip—and you'll need to accommodate it. Resist the impulse to rush to catch up and try retreating a week on the charts. To double-check on whether you're overexerting yourself, refer to the guidelines on personal stress and recovery heart and breathing rates, pages 50-51.

WARMING UP

You wouldn't think of starting your car in winter without warming it up first, would you? Your muscles and joints should have the same preliminary conditioning before you exercise them. Sometimes I do a slow jog to warm up before running and lately I've been limbering up with Jack La-Lanne on television in the morning while I'm still in my pajamas. Then I do my laps.

If you're over 40, Ken suggests a slow 3-minute walk for warming up. Younger women may like to preface their exercise with calisthenics, which are good not only as warm-ups, but also to enhance coordination and graceful movement.

Aerobics-cum-Calisthenics

Calisthenics, as we said in Chapter 4, are a fine supplement to aerobics but in no way a substitute. They make no contribution to cardiovascular fitness, though they're definitely good warm-ups.

Prior to exercise, Ken recommends working up to 20 repetitions of each of these 5 basic calisthenics (they're also used by women members of the United States Marine Corps).

1. *Trunk circling:* Stand with your legs apart and twist the upper part of your body alternately to the left and the right, rotating mainly from the waist.

2. *Toe touching:* With your legs fairly close together, bend from the waist to touch your toes with outstretched

arms. If you can't reach all the way down with your knees straight, bend your knees slightly.

3. *Side leg-raise:* Lie on the floor on your side and raise your leg from the hip, then lower it again. Repeat this about 10 times, then turn to the other side and raise and lower your other leg 10 times.

4. *Sit-ups:* Lie on the floor, on your back, with your knees bent. Raise your trunk to a sitting position without the help of your arms, then lie down again *slowly*. Start with about 10 repetitions. (Sit-ups are traditionally attempted with legs stretched out flat against the floor. Ken advises against this because the stress on your knees and back may cause pain and even injury. It's far safer to bend your knees slightly.)

5. *Side bends:* Stand with your feet apart and extend your arms above your head with fingertips touching. Bend slowly sideways from your waist—as far as possible. Keep your arms straight and don't bend your elbows. Remain bent sideways for several seconds. Then straighten up and make a similar bend to the other side, again holding the bent position for a few seconds.

COOLING DOWN

A tapering-off period after exercise is just as vital as the warming up beforehand. I do it by strolling around our yard and maybe pulling weeds for 5 minutes. Whatever *you* do, resist that impulse to flop!

If you don't heed this precaution, you risk dizziness and even fainting. In particular, avoid going from a cool temperature to a warm one right away, or vice versa. This would also increase your tendency to faint. Especially after running, don't sit down immediately, but keep in motion for a short time. Running causes blood to pool in your legs and unless you give it a chance to get back to your heart and brain in sufficient quantity, you could black out.

By the time you've cooled down, you may be ready for that refreshing (and low-calorie) piece of fresh fruit or glass of iced tea. And lady, you are certainly going to feel vigorous, virtuous and victorious.

FALLING OFF

I'd be unrealistic if I didn't acknowledge that all of us occasionally have lapses in our good intentions about exercise. I do. I'm awfully good at finding those elaborate, unacceptable excuses, especially when I'm traveling with Ken on his lecture tours. (And that's when we're eating at banquet after banquet, too.)

If you do drop out, please make it temporary. Don't be so demoralized that you get melodramatic and say "Goodbye forever" to your exercise program.

Be human. Forgive yourself and start again. In fact, turn the page and start *now*, whether it's your first start or your fortieth.

8: The Aerobics Chart Pack for Women

1. Read Chapters 4, 6 and 7 thoroughly before you start one of the following age-adjusted progressive exercise programs.
2. After observing any medical precautions specified, select an exercise program compatible with your age.

If you are:	*Your exercise programs are on pages:*
Under 30	64–67
30–39	68–71
40–49	71–74
50–59	75–79
Over 60	79–82

3. After you've completed the basic program, continue to earn at least 24 points a week—either in the exercise program you conditioned yourself in or by combining various exercises to achieve the minimum points.

RUNNING EXERCISE PROGRAM
(under 30 years of age)

WEEK	DISTANCE (miles)	TIME GOAL (minutes)	FREQ/WK	POINTS/WK
1	1	17:00	5	5
2	1	15:00	5	5
3	1½	23:00	5	7½
4	1½	21:00	5	15
5	1	10:30	5	15
6	1½	19:00	5	15
7	1½	18:00	5	15
8	2	24:00	5	20
9	1½	14:30	4	24
10	1½	13:30	4	24

NOTE   First 4 weeks are walking only.

WALKING EXERCISE PROGRAM
(under 30 years of age)

WEEK	DISTANCE (miles)	TIME GOAL (minutes)	FREQ/WK	POINTS/WK
1	1	18:00	5	5
2	1	16:00	5	5
3	1½	25:00	5	7½
4	1½	23:00	5	7½
5	1	13:45	5	10
6	2	29:30	5	10
7	1½	21:30	5	15
8	2	28:30	5	20
9	2	27:30	5	20
10	2½	35:00	5	25

ROPE SKIPPING EXERCISE PROGRAM
(under 30 years of age)

WEEK	DURATION (minutes)	FREQ/WK	POINTS/WK
1	2:30	5	—
2	5:00	5	7½
3	5:00	5	7½
4	7:30	5	11¼
5	7:30	5	11¼
6	10:00	5	15
7	12:30	5	18¾
8	14:00	5	21⅔
9	15:00	5	22½
10	16:00	5	26¼

NOTE Skip with both feet together or step over the rope, alternating feet, skipping at a frequency of 70-80 steps per minute.

STAIR CLIMBING EXERCISE PROGRAM

(under 30 years of age)

WEEK	ROUND TRIPS (average number per minute)	DURATION (minutes)	FREQ/WK	POINTS/WK
1	5	2:00	5	—
2	5	4:00	5	—
3	6	6:30	5	7½
4	6	7:30	5	8¾
5	6	9:45	5	11
6	7	9:00	5	15
7	7	10:30	5	17½
8	7	12:00	5	20
9	8	10:00	5	22
10	8	11:00	5	25

NOTE Applies to 10 steps, 6"–7" in height, 25°–30° incline. Use of banister is encouraged.

SWIMMING EXERCISE PROGRAM

(under 30 years of age)

WEEK	DISTANCE (yards)	TIME GOAL (minutes)	FREQ/WK	POINTS/WK
1	100	3:00	5	—
2	150	3:45	5	—
3	200	5:00	5	7½
4	200	4:30	5	7½
5	250	5:30	5	10
6	300	7:00	5	12½
7	400	8:30	5	17½
8	500	11:00	5	20
9	550	12:00	5	22½
10	600	13:00	5	25

CYCLING EXERCISE PROGRAM
(under 30 years of age)

WEEK	DISTANCE (miles)	TIME GOAL (minutes)	FREQ/WK	POINTS/WK
1	2.0	12:30	5	—
2	2.0	11:00	5	5
3	2.0	9:45	5	5
4	3.0	16:00	5	7½
5	3.0	14:30	5	7½
6	4.0	20:00	5	10
7	5.0	25:00	5	12½
8	6.0	30:00	5	15
9	7.0	35:00	4	22
10	8.0	40:00	4	26

STATIONARY CYCLING EXERCISE PROGRAM
(under 30 years of age)

WEEK	CYCLING SPEED (m.p.h.)	DURATION (minutes)	*PR after exercise	FREQ/WK	POINTS/WK
1	12	5:00	130	5	5
2	12	7:30	130	5	5
3	12	10:00	140	5	5
4	15	12:30	140	5	7½
5	15	16:00	140	5	10
6	15	18:00	140	5	11¼
7	17½	21:00	150	5	15
8	20	21:00	150	5	20
9	20	24:00	150	5	22½
10	20	27:00	150	5	25

NOTE Add enough resistance that the pulse rate (PR), counted for 10 seconds immediately after exercise and multiplied by 6, equals the number specified. If it is higher, lower the resistance before cycling again; if it is lower, increase the resistance.

RUNNING EXERCISE PROGRAM
(30–39 years of age)

WEEK	DISTANCE (miles)	TIME GOAL (minutes)	FREQ/WK	POINTS/WK
1	1	18:30	5	5
2	1	16:30	5	5
3	1	15:30	5	5
4	1½	24:00	5	7½
5	1½	22:00	5	7½
6	1	12:00	5	10
7	1½	20:00	5	15
8	1½	18:00	5	15
9	2	25:00	5	20
10	2	24:00	5	20
11	1½	16:00	5	22
12	1½	14:00	4	24

NOTE First 5 weeks are walking only.

WALKING EXERCISE PROGRAM
(30–39 years of age)

WEEK	DISTANCE (miles)	TIME GOAL (minutes)	FREQ/WK	POINTS/WK
1	1	19:00	5	5
2	1	17:00	5	5
3	1	15:30	5	5
4	1½	26:00	5	7½
5	1½	23:30	5	7½
6	1	14:15	5	10
7	2	31:00	5	10
8	2	30:00	5	10
9	1½	21:30	5	15
10	2	28:45	5	20
11	2	28:00	5	20
12	2½	35:30	5	25

ROPE SKIPPING EXERCISE PROGRAM
(30–39 years of age)

WEEK	DURATION (minutes)	FREQ/WK	POINTS/WK
1	2:30	5	—
2	2:30	5	—
3	5:00	5	7½
4	5:00	5	7½
5	7:30	5	11¼
6	7:30	5	11¼
7	10:00	5	15
8	11:00	5	16⅔
9	12:00	5	18⅓
10	13:00	5	20
11	15:00	5	22½
12	16:00	5	26¼

NOTE   Skip with both feet together or step over the rope, alternating feet, skipping at a frequency of 70–80 steps per minute.

STAIR CLIMBING EXERCISE PROGRAM
(30–39 years of age)

WEEK	ROUND TRIPS (average number per minute)	DURATION (minutes)	FREQ/WK	POINTS/WK
1	5	2:00	5	—
2	5	3:00	5	—
3	5	4:00	5	—
4	6	5:00	5	5
5	6	6:30	5	7½
6	6	7:30	5	8¾
7	6	8:30	5	10
8	7	7:00	5	11¼
9	7	8:00	5	13¾
10	7	9:00	5	15
11	8	10:00	5	22½
12	8	11:00	5	25

NOTE   Applies to 10 steps, 6"–7" in height, 20°–30° incline. Use of banister is encouraged.

SWIMMING EXERCISE PROGRAM

(30–39 years of age)

WEEK	DISTANCE (yards)	TIME GOAL (minutes)	FREQ/WK	POINTS/WK
1	100	3:15	5	—
2	150	4:00	5	—
3	150	3:45	5	—
4	200	4.30	5	7½
5	250	5:45	5	10
6	250	5:30	5	10
7	300	7:15	5	12½
8	350	8:00	5	15
9	400	9:00	5	17½
10	450	9:30	5	20
11	500	11:30	5	20
12	600	13:30	5	25

CYCLING EXERCISE PROGRAM

(30–39 years of age)

WEEK	DISTANCE (miles)	TIME GOAL (minutes)	FREQ/WK	POINTS/WK
1	2	13:00	5	—
2	2	12:00	5	—
3	2	10:00	5	5
4	3	17:00	5	7½
5	3	15:00	5	7½
6	4	22:00	5	10
7	4	21:00	5	10
8	5	26:00	5	12½
9	5	25:30	5	12½
10	6	31:00	5	15
11	7	36:00	4	22
12	8	42:00	4	26

STATIONARY CYCLING EXERCISE PROGRAM
(30–39 years of age)

WEEK	CYCLING SPEED (m.p.h.)	DURATION (minutes)	*PR after exercise	FREQ/WK	POINTS/WK
1	10	5:00	125	5	—
2	10	7:30	125	5	—
3	12	7:30	130	5	—
4	12	10:00	130	5	5
5	12	12:30	130	5	6¼
6	15	12:30	140	5	7½
7	15	12:30	140	5	7½
8	17½	14:00	140	5	10
9	17½	16:00	145	5	11¼
10	20	17:30	150	5	17½
11	20	21:00	150	5	20
12	20	27:00	150	5	25

NOTE   Add enough resistance that the pulse rate (PR), counted for 10 seconds immediately after exercise and multiplied by 6, equals the number specified. If it is higher, lower the resistance before cycling again; if it is lower, increase the resistance.

RUNNING EXERCISE PROGRAM
(40–49 years of age)

WEEK	DISTANCE (miles)	TIME GOAL (minutes)	FREQ/WK	POINTS/WK
1	1	19:00	5	5
2	1	17:30	5	5
3	1	16:00	5	5
4	1½	25:00	5	7½
5	1½	23:00	5	7½
6	2	31:00	5	10
7	1	12:30	5	10
8	1½	20:30	5	15
9	1½	19:00	5	15
10	2	26:00	5	20
11	2	24:00	5	20
12	1½	17:00	5	22
13	1½	15:30	5	22
14	1½	<14:30	4	24

NOTE   First 6 weeks are walking only.

WALKING EXERCISE PROGRAM
(40–49 years of age)

WEEK	DISTANCE (miles)	TIME GOAL (minutes)	FREQ/WK	POINTS/WK
1	1	20:00	5	—
2	1	18:00	5	5
3	1	16:00	5	5
4	1	15:00	5	5
5	1½	27:00	5	7½
6	1½	26:00	5	7½
7	1½	25:00	5	7½
8	1	14:25	5	10
9	2	33:00	5	10
10	2	32:00	5	10
11	1½	21:40	5	15
12	2	28:50	5	20
13	2	28:30	5	20
14	2½	36:00	5	25

ROPE SKIPPING EXERCISE PROGRAM
(40–49 years of age)

WEEK	DURATION (minutes)	FREQ/WK	POINTS/WK
1	2:00	5	—
2	2:30	5	—
3	5:00	5	7½
4	5:00	5	7½
5	5:00	5	7½
6	7:30	5	11¼
7	10:00	5	15
8	10:00	5	15
9	11:00	5	16⅔
10	11:00	5	16⅔
11	12:00	5	18⅓
12	13:00	5	20
13	14:00	5	21⅔
14	10:00 (in A.M.) and 7:00 (in P.M.)	5	25

NOTE   Skip with both feet together or step over the rope, alternating feet, skipping at a frequency of 70–80 steps per minute.

STAIR CLIMBING EXERCISE PROGRAM
(40–49 years of age)

WEEK	ROUND TRIPS (average number per minute)	DURATION (minutes)	FREQ/WK	POINTS/WK
1	5	1:00	5	—
2	5	2:00	5	—
3	5	3:00	5	—
4	5	4:00	5	—
5	6	5:00	5	5
6	6	6:30	5	7½
7	6	7:30	5	8¾
8	6	8:30	5	10
9	6	9:45	5	11¼
10	6	11:00	5	12½
11	6	6:30 (in A.M.) 6:30 (in P.M.)	5	15
12	6	7:30 (in A.M.) 7:30 (in P.M.)	5	17½
13	7	7:00 (in A.M.) 7:00 (in P.M.)	5	22½
14	7	9:00 (in A.M.) 6:00 (in P.M.)	5	25

NOTE Applies to 10 steps, 6"–7" in height, 25°–30° incline. Use of banister is encouraged.

SWIMMING EXERCISE PROGRAM
(40–49 years of age)

WEEK	DISTANCE (yards)	TIME GOAL (minutes)	FREQ/WK	POINTS/WK
1	100	3:30	4	—
2	100	3:15	5	—
3	150	4:30	5	—
4	150	4:00	5	—
5	200	5:15	5	5
6	250	6:00	5	10
7	300	7:15	5	12½
8	300	7:00	5	12½
9	350	8:15	5	15
10	400	9:30	5	17½
11	450	10:00	5	20
12	500	11:45	5	20
13	550	12:15	5	22½
14	600	14:00	5	25

CYCLING EXERCISE PROGRAM
(40–49 years of age)

WEEK	DISTANCE (miles)	TIME GOAL (minutes)	FREQ/WK	POINTS/WK
1	2	13:30	5	—
2	2	12:30	5	—
3	2	10:30	5	5
4	3	17:30	5	7½
5	3	15:30	5	7½
6	4	23:30	5	10
7	4	22:00	5	10
8	5	27:00	5	12½
9	5	26:00	5	12½
10	6	33:00	5	15
11	6	32:00	5	15
12	7	38:00	4	22
13	7	37:00	4	22
14	8	44:00	4	26

STATIONARY CYCLING EXERCISE PROGRAM
(40–49 years of age)

WEEK	CYCLING SPEED (m.p.h.)	DURATION (minutes)	*PR after exercise	FREQ/WK	POINTS/WK
1	10	5:00	120	5	—
2	10	5:00	120	5	—
3	10	7:30	125	5	—
4	12	7:30	125	5	—
5	12	10:00	130	5	5
6	12	12:30	130	5	6¼
7	15	12:30	130	5	7½
8	15	12:30	130	5	7½
9	17½	15:00	135	5	10⅜
10	17½	15:00	135	5	10⅜
11	17½	17:30	140	5	12½
12	20	17:30	140	5	17½
13	20	21:00	145	5	20
14	20	27:00	145	5	25

NOTE Add enough resistance that the pulse rate (PR), counted for 10 seconds immediately after exercise and multiplied by 6, equals the number specified. If it is higher, lower the resistance before cycling again; if it is lower, increase the resistance.

RUNNING EXERCISE PROGRAM
(50–59 years of age)

WEEK	DISTANCE (miles)	TIME GOAL (minutes)	FREQ/WK	POINTS/WK
1	1	20:00	5	—
2	1	18:00	5	5
3	1	17:00	5	5
4	1	16:00	5	5
5	1½	26:00	5	7½
6	1½	24:00	5	7½
7	1½	23:00	5	7½
8	2	32:00	5	10
9	1	13:00	5	10
10	1½	20:00	5	15
11	1½	18:00	5	15
12	2	28:00	5	20
13	2	26:00	5	20
14	1½	17:30	5	22
15	1½	17:00	5	22
16	1½	16:30	5	22

NOTE First 8 weeks are walking only.

WALKING EXERCISE PROGRAM
(50–59 years of age)

WEEK	DISTANCE (miles)	TIME GOAL (minutes)	FREQ/WK	POINTS/WK
1	¾	18:00	5	—
2	1	25:00	5	—
3	1	22:00	5	—
4	1	20:00	5	—
5	1	18:00	5	5
6	1½	28:00	5	7½
7	1½	27:00	5	7½
8	1½	26:00	5	7½
9	2	34:00	5	10
10	2	33:00	5	10
11	2	32:00	5	10
12	2½	40:00	5	12½
13	2½	38:00	5	12½
14	3	46:00	5	15½
15	3	45:00	6	18
16	3	43:15	4	24

ROPE SKIPPING EXERCISE PROGRAM
(50–59 years of age)

WEEK	DURATION (minutes)	FREQ/WK	POINTS/WK
1	1:30	5	—
2	2:30	5	—
3	2:30	5	—
4	5:00	5	7½
5	5:00	5	7½
6	5:00	5	7½
7	6:00	5	8⅓
8	7:00	5	10
9	8:00	5	11⅔
10	9:00	5	13⅓
11	10:00	5	15
12	11:00	5	16⅔
13	12:00	5	18⅓
14	13:00	5	20
15	14:00	5	21⅔
16	10:00 (in A.M.) and 7:00 (in P.M.)	5	25

NOTE   Skip with both feet together or step over the rope, alternating feet, skipping at a frequency of 70–80 steps per minute.

STAIR CLIMBING EXERCISE PROGRAM
(50–59 years of age)

WEEK	ROUND TRIPS (average number per minute)	DURATION (minutes)	FREQ/WK	POINTS/WK
1	4	2:00	5	—
2	5	1:00	5	—
3	5	2:00	5	—
4	5	3:00	5	—
5	5	4:00	5	—
6	5	5:00	5	2½
7	5	6:00	5	3¾
8	5	7:00	5	5
9	5	9:00	5	7½
10	5	11:00	5	10
11	5	12:00	5	11½
12	6	11:00	5	12½
13	6	12:00	5	13¾
14	6	13:00	5	15
15	6	7:30 (in A.M.) 7:30 (in P.M.)	5	17½
16	6	8:30 (in A.M.) 8:30 (in P.M.)	5	20
17	6	10:00 (in A.M.) 10:00 (in P.M.)	5	22½
18	6	12:00 (in A.M.) 10:00 (in P.M.)	5	25

NOTE   Applies to 10 steps, 6"–7" in height, 25°–30° incline. Use of banister is encouraged.

SWIMMING EXERCISE PROGRAM
(50–59 years of age)

WEEK	DISTANCE (yards)	TIME GOAL (minutes)	FREQ/WK	POINTS/WK
1	50	2:00	3	—
2	100	4:00	4	—
3	100	3:30	5	—
4	150	5:15	5	—
5	150	5:00	5	—
6	200	6:00	5	5
7	250	7:00	5	6¼
8	250	6:30	5	6¼
9	300	8:00	5	7½
10	300	7:30	5	12½
11	350	8:30	5	15
12	400	9:55	5	17½
13	450	11:00	5	20
14	500	12:00	5	20
15	550	13:00	5	22½
16	600	14:30	5	25

CYCLING EXERCISE PROGRAM
(50–59 years of age)

WEEK	DISTANCE (miles)	TIME GOAL (minutes)	FREQ/WK	POINTS/WK
1	2	14:00	5	—
2	2	13:00	5	—
3	2	11:00	5	5
4	3	17:45	5	7½
5	3	16:00	5	7½
6	3	15:30	5	7½
7	4	23:45	5	10
8	4	23:00	5	10
9	5	28:00	5	12½
10	5	27:00	5	12½
11	6	34:00	5	15
12	6	33:00	5	15
13	7	40:00	4	22
14	7	38:00	4	22
15	8	47:00	4	26
16	8	46:00	4	26

STATIONARY CYCLING EXERCISE PROGRAM

(50–59 years of age)

WEEK	CYCLING SPEED (m.p.h.)	DURATION (minutes)	*PR after exercise	FREQ/WK	POINTS/WK
1	10	5:00	120	5	—
2	10	5:00	120	5	—
3	12	5:00	120	5	—
4	12	7:30	125	5	—
5	15	7:30	125	5	—
6	15	10:00	125	5	6¼
7	15	12:30	130	5	7½
8	15	14:00	130	5	8¾
9	15	16:00	130	5	10
10	17½	16:00	130	5	11¼
11	17½	17:30	130	5	12½
12	17½	21:00	135	5	15
13	20	17:30	135	5	17½
14	20	21:00	140	5	20
15	20	22:30	140	5	22½
16	20	27:00	140	5	25

NOTE Add enough resistance that the pulse rate (PR), counted for 10 seconds immediately after exercise and multiplied by 6, equals the number specified. If it is higher, lower the resistance before cycling again; if it is lower, increase the resistance.

RUNNING EXERCISE PROGRAM

(over 60 years of age)

Not recommended.

WALKING EXERCISE PROGRAM
(over 60 years of age)

WEEK	DISTANCE (miles)	TIME GOAL (minutes)	FREQ/WK	POINTS/WK
1	½	13:00	5	—
2	¾	20:00	5	—
3	1	26:00	5	—
4	1	25:00	5	—
5	1	24:00	5	—
6	1	22:00	5	—
7	1	20:00	5	5
8	1½	32:00	5	—
9	1½	30:00	5	—
10	1½	28:00	5	7½
11	2	38:00	5	—
12	2	36:00	5	—
13	2	34:00	5	10
14	2½	45:00	5	12½
15	2½	44:00	5	12½
16	2½	43:00	5	12½
17	3	52:00	5	15
18	3	50:00	5	15

ROPE SKIPPING EXERCISE PROGRAM
(over 60 years of age)
Not recommended.

STAIR CLIMBING EXERCISE PROGRAM
(over 60 years of age)
Not recommended.

SWIMMING EXERCISE PROGRAM
(over 60 years of age)

WEEK	DISTANCE (yards)	TIME GOAL (minutes)	FREQ/WK	POINTS/WK
1	50	2:30	3	—
2	50	2:00	4	—
3	100	4:30	4	—
4	100	4:00	5	—
5	150	5:30	5	—
6	200	7:00	5	—
7	200	6:30	5	5
8	250	7:15	5	6¼
9	250	7:00	5	6¼
10	300	9:00	5	7½
11	300	8:30	5	7½
12	350	9:00	5	10
13	400	10:30	5	12½
14	450	11:30	5	15
15	450	11:10	5	20
16	500	12:25	5	20
17	550	13:30	5	22½
18	600	< 15:00	5	25

CYCLING EXERCISE PROGRAM
(over 60 years of age)

WEEK	DISTANCE (miles)	TIME GOAL (minutes)	FREQ/WK	POINTS/WK
1	1	10:00	5	—
2	1	8:00	5	—
3	2	16:00	5	—
4	2	14:00	5	—
5	2	11:30	5	5
6	3	17:45	5	7½
7	3	17:30	5	7½
8	3	17:00	5	7½
9	4	25:00	5	10
10	4	24:30	5	10
11	4	24:00	5	10
12	5	29:30	5	12½
13	5	29:00	5	12½
14	5	28:30	5	12½
15	5	28:00	5	12½
16	6	35:30	5	15
17	6	35:00	5	15
18	6	34:00	5	15

NOTE Three-wheeled cycling is encouraged.

STATIONARY CYCLING EXERCISE PROGRAM

(over 60 years of age)

WEEK	CYCLING SPEED (m.p.h.)	DURATION (minutes)	*PR after exercise	FREQ/WK	POINTS/WK
1	10	2:30	100	5	—
2	10	3:30	100	5	—
3	10	5:00	110	5	—
4	12	5:00	110	5	—
5	12	7:30	110	5	—
6	12	7:30	110	5	—
7	15	7:30	110	5	—
8	15	10:00	115	5	—
9	15	12:00	115	5	7
10	15	12:30	120	5	7½
11	15	16:00	120	5	10
12	15	18:00	120	5	11¼
13	17½	16:00	125	5	10
14	17½	16:00	125	5	11¼
15	17½	17:30	130	5	12½
16	20	14:00	130	5	15
17	20	17:30	130	5	17½
18	20	21:00	130	5	20

NOTE   Add enough resistance that the pulse rate (PR), counted for 10 seconds immediately after exercise and multiplied by 6, equals the number specified. If it is higher, lower the resistance before cycling again; if it is lower, increase the resistance.

9: Use Guide for Outdoor Aerobic Exercise

IN INTRODUCING YOU to aerobics, I've borne in mind the well-known story about the little schoolgirl whose book report consisted of one sentence: "This told me more than I wanted to know about the subject of penguins." I realize that many readers are familiar with Ken's earlier books on aerobics, and with the great care he has taken to report and document every step of his research and tests relating to cardiovascular conditioning. So my approach has been to sketch, rather than itemize, the scientific background, the years of conducting projects and studies that authenticate the value of aerobics. I've concentrated on trying to explain clearly but concisely the results and benefits of this kind of exercise as they pertain to women.

Most of all, I've wanted to persuade you to sample aerobics. When you feel you have something great going in your life, you're compelled to share it, to tell the world. I am, anyway. (I remember when I started college—coming from a very small town in Oklahoma, graduating in a high school class of 17—I was so excited, so overwhelmed by that tremendous world of knowledge that I'd come home and keep my parents up for hours at night talking about it. I was so stimulated by what I was learning that I *had* to pass it along.)

Now you know what the broad aerobics program is, how it works and why it's effective, and you've seen the Aerobics Chart Pack for Women with its wonderfully varied "carte du jour." Here and in the next chapter I'll be more specific about Ken's recommendations for using the individual programs, and about what you can expect when you get involved in them—outdoor exercises first, and then ones you do indoors.

NEOPHYTE EXERCISERS

As you looked through the chart pack, you saw that each exercise program is progressive, age-adjusted and has a built-in orientation designed to prepare your body gradually for full aerobic conditioning. *If you haven't been in the habit of exercising on a regular basis, under no circumstances should you take any one of the fitness tests on pages 52-54.* This rule is especially important if you're over 30 and if you haven't had the type of medical examination specified on page 43.

Once you've completed the basic program, you have the option of taking the fitness test of your choice. If the results of the test put you in Category IV (Good) or Category V (Excellent), you have the satisfaction of knowing you have only to maintain your present level of fitness.

HABITUAL EXERCISERS

If you've been in the habit of exercising consistently—say, as a minimum standard, 3 times a week for the past 6 weeks —and if you've had the form of medical checkup indicated for your age category, you're free to pinpoint your fitness level immediately by taking any one of the fitness tests. If you place in Categories I, II, or III (Very Poor, Poor or Fair), assign yourself to one of the exercise programs in the chart pack and follow it through; if you placed in Categories IV or V, just keep up the good work.

THE GREAT, GRATIFYING OUTDOORS

Personally, I don't have any ax to grind for outdoor exercise over indoor, or vice versa. But I can't resist including a short commercial on the joy of working out in the open air.

Pediatricians wax eloquent on the benefits of fresh air

and sunshine for infants, and any mother who's had the experience of putting a fretful baby out in the yard in a carriage or playpen knows that simply being outdoors often acts as an instant tranquilizer for tiny fussbudgets. Also, the mild "jogging" action of being wheeled in a carriage or carried in a baby sling or parents' arms as they walk seems to soothe babies.

Without making a scientific case of it, I suggest that for adults the combination of motion and exposure to fresh air is also a natural tonic for mind and body. It amounts to a kind of sensitivity training, too, in that as you experience the warmth of the sun or the brisk massage of the wind, your eyes begin to see more, your ears and nose to discern more, your body to respond more to what it feels and perceives from the natural elements.

If you exercise in the open air, open your senses to the scenery, the weather, the pleasure of the now. Discover that aesthetics and athletics are not incompatible.

WALKING PROGRAM

I'm sure many women will prefer this less vigorous method of conditioning. It *does* consume more time per session, but it has the overwhelming advantage of being feasible for anyone, anytime, anyplace. It doesn't even have to look like exercise. For those of you who are self-conscious, the latter can make a decisive difference. Also, it's an easy way to pick up points. You can make it part of your routine (by walking to the store, the office, the kids' school) without its ever seeming like a routine.

Few cautionary notes are called for if your aerobics choice is walking. If you follow the progressive program meticulously, you're not likely to have any trouble. Naturally, you'd be wise to wear practical, well-fitted shoes with low heels and good support. And you'll find it helpful to read the next section, on running, which discusses foot and leg physiology. Remember, though walking may seem the least strenuous of the exercise programs, if you're not used to doing it on a prolonged, daily basis, you'll be "feeling it" till the training effect takes over.

RUNNING PROGRAM

Like walking, running is versatile. You can do it alone or in groups, indoors or out and at any time of day. It exercises the arms as well as the legs, has a firming effect on muscle groups throughout the body, especially the abdomen, and it's the quickest way to get the training effect started.

Occasionally women ask me, "How do you breathe when you run?" My answer: Any way I can. If you allow yourself to become self-conscious about breathing—trying to inhale when your right foot comes down and so on—you'll be uncomfortable. It's like becoming aware of your tongue in your mouth. Pretty soon it gets so awkward you can't stand it—you think, "Do I have to live with this the rest of my life?" I try my best not to think about what I'm doing when I exercise. I tune out the physical presence of my body and what it's doing and concentrate on the scenery or let my mind wander to my plans for the rest of the day.

Actually, questions about foot, leg and back sensitivity are much more frequent, and appropriate, because these are the areas in which running is most likely to create a reaction. For example, many women develop foot problems during the initial stages of a running program. Typical ones include swollen ankles, tendonitis (affecting the Achilles tendon, which connects your heel and calf—it becomes sore and inflamed) and "jogger's heel," which results from pounding away on hard pavements. Three factors are important in avoiding these conditions: the right shoes, the right running or jogging surface and the right running or jogging style.

The right footgear, as I described it in Chapter 6, has a thick cushioned or rippled sole, arch support and a little heel—the cost ranges between $15 and $20. With proper arch and heel support, you reduce your chances of having tendon problems and ankle soreness and you enhance your general comfort when running.

The right surface is smooth and resilient—grass, dirt or

a well-kept running track are ideal. However, since pavement is much more plentiful than any of these, you'll probably have to ask your shoes to do the whole job of cushioning. You can see why we urge you to invest in a special pair just for exercise.

The right style makes the difference between accomplishment and disappointment, ease and difficulty, for a runner. Ken's advice is that you use the classic style, in which you run almost flat-footed. Let the heel of your foot strike the ground a little ahead of the rest of your foot, then roll gently forward on the ball of the foot. If you hit too hard on the soft tissue of your heel, you'll end up with jogger's heel. If you go to the other extreme and get up on your toes and do primary springing, you're making yourself vulnerable to an injury of the Achilles tendon. As for the rest of your body, don't bounce and don't tighten your knees—if they're slightly flexed, they cushion some of the pell-mell impact of your running. Your arms should follow the movement of your body, swinging easily at your sides.

If, after observing these precautions, you still develop sore ankles or feet, Ken's rule is: Stop exercising if this activity makes the pain worse; otherwise, continue with caution—running at slower speeds and for shorter distances. In most cases, if you continue to exercise slowly, even with pain in your ankles, the soreness disappears. Personally, I've found I get over my soreness much faster if I continue to exercise at a more moderate pace than if I stop completely. I compare it to plucking my eyebrows. It hurts, but it's transient and I like the results.

The knees, legs and back are occasionally the source of problems for runners. Shin splints—soreness in muscles below the knee—are fairly common. The usual cause is running on hard surfaces in hard shoes and the cure is switching to resilient surfaces and flexible, cushioned shoes. Knee and joint soreness may turn up in women with a history of arthritis or old knee injuries. Leg muscles may tend to cramp before they become fully conditioned, but these spasms are likely to disappear as you continue your exercise.

CYCLING

Here you do need a special piece of equipment, and reasonably favorable weather conditions to pursue the program—obviously wintry and windy days aren't conducive to cycling. But if wherewithal and weather aren't problems for you, cycling can become part of your life in an unobtrusive and enjoyable way. Use your bike alone or in groups, for transportation to the office, shops or informal social events. And don't forget the ecological benefits of biking!

As with walking, aside from "feeling it" when you're beginning to exercise on a bicycle, this kind of conditioning is almost free of typical complaints. Almost any type of cycle—3 speeds or less or a tri-wheeler—is suitable for aerobic exercise and the type you use doesn't appreciably affect the point values given in the charts.

SWIMMING

If you don't have a fear or dislike of water (as I do), and have access to a suitable pool or swimming area (in cities, check out YM/WCA facilities or health clubs), this form of exercise will provide superb aerobic benefits to your internal organs and muscles.

No particular cautions here, either. If you're a swimmer, you're probably already aware of any problems that are likely to arise for you as an individual, such as eye, ear or nose troubles. But apart from avoiding overexertion and undue fatigue—something you should guard against in any form of exercise—you should find your swimming program trouble-free.

That covers the exercises that are essentially done outdoors (I realize that all *can* conceivably be done inside, too, but for the sake of simplicity I've separated them from those you would normally do indoors). In the next chapter, stationary running and cycling, running on a treadmill, rope skipping and stair climbing are profiled—as well as special equipment where it's called for.

10: Inside Tips on Aerobic Exercise and Equipment

MORE WOMEN THAN men exercise indoors. Probably the chief reason is necessity (for mothers who are housebound with young children); other factors are convenience and, for many, I'm sure, a desire for privacy. The last reason is just as real and valid as the other two. Some women simply feel undignified astride a bicycle or loping along public thoroughfares. For them, exercising inside seems more natural and comfortable. Why not? The choice is wide and the conditioning is just as effective. As for the modes of indoor exercise, the first one I want to bring up is the source of some controversy in the Cooper household.

STATIONARY RUNNING

Running in place is very popular with women and the appeal, I think, is that it's easy to do and easy to persist in. Ken thinks it's not so easy, harder on the feet and ankles than normal running, and tedious as well. You'll have to judge for yourself. It may not be as glamorous to say you can run in place for 15 minutes as it is to say you can run 2 miles, but I know from many, many letters and conversations with women that they like and use this form of aerobic conditioning—both as an everyday exercise and as a substitute on days when weather or busyness makes it impossible to get out of the house to do other forms of exercise.

In any case, stationary running is recommended only for the premenopausal woman (see chart in the Appendix, page 153). When the change of life has occurred, our sex in particular is more susceptible to weakening or decalcification of the bones, and the chance of a foot fracture is increased.

To avoid foot and ankle problems, the younger woman who chooses running in place as "her" exercise should resist the temptation to do it barefoot. That's just asking for trouble. You need the support and cushioning of a jogging shoe to prevent soreness and tendonitis. Second, always run on a resilient surface rather than the hard floor. A soft, thick rug with an underliner is fine, or you can buy a small sponge-rubber pad just for stationary running. Remember, you've got to raise each foot a minimum of 8 inches off the floor and achieve a minimum of 60 steps a minute to begin earning points. To estimate your rate of steps per minute, count each time your left foot hits the floor for 15 seconds, then multiply by 4.

To beat boredom, some women tell me they listen to the radio or watch television as they run in place. Ken has also worked out variations on stationary running that you might want to use to make the basic routine more interesting.

One Step Up Using a step with carpeting or a rubber tread to prevent slipping, step up and down rapidly at the rate of 30 to 40 cycles a minute. Start with both feet on the floor, put one foot on the step, then the other—don't jump—then one down, then the other. The following chart spells out aerobic point values for this variation.

ONE STEP UP (7″) POINT CHART

STEPPING RATE (per min.)	TIME (min.)	POINTS
30	6:30	1½
	9:45	2¼
	13:00	3
35	6:00	2
	9:00	3
	12:00	4
40	5:00	2½
	7:30	3¾
	10:00	5

Three Steps Up Here you run up and down 3 steps, turning around on the third so you face forward coming down. The point value for 20 round trips a minute is about equal to that for running in place at the rate of 70 to 80 steps a minute. Twenty-five to 30 round trips a minute would approximate the point value for stationary running at 80 to 90 steps a minute. The main problem here is dizziness.

ROPE SKIPPING

Ken feels that rope skipping is much more appropriate and comfortable for women than stationary running because it involves enough forward movement to take the impact off a purely vertical plane. In consequence, the danger of foot, leg and ankle pain is lessened. It's also a little more physiological than running in place in that the muscles of your arms, shoulders and upper body get more of a workout, thus more toning action. (However, like swimming, it does involve a skill factor—you have to be coordinated.)

Jump with both feet together, or step over the rope alternating feet. The rate should be 70 to 80 skips a minute.

STAIR CLIMBING

To tell you the truth, this form of exercise—a perfectly good one aerobically speaking, if done properly—didn't occur to Ken as a possibility when he wrote his first book on aerobics. Being Southwesterners, we're used to one-level ranch-style houses and we're less aware of stairways in general. After the book came out, we got dozens of letters asking if stair climbing could be evaluated aerobically. It certainly can—it's like a built-in aerobics track for people who live in two-story houses or apartment buildings. But the trick lies in sustaining the effort long enough to exercise your heart and lungs sufficiently to create a significant oxygen debt. That is, you have to counteract the rest you get when you go down the stairs.

The 3-step-up cycle described in the section on stationary running provides enough continuity in your energy output to earn aerobic points. So do the programs Ken worked out for a 10-step flight of stairs given in Chapter 8.

Again, it's good insurance to wear shoes that give your feet both cushioning and support and to hold on to the banisters.

STATIONARY CYCLING

My impression is that exercise on a stationary bicycle—a permanently mounted piece of equipment with handlebars, a seat, pedals and one wheel—is really coming on strong with women. It has numerous advantages besides proximity, convenience and privacy. The bike can be used by all the family (great physiotherapy for the elderly). It can be set up unobtrusively in the corner of a room, makes a fine birthday, holiday or anniversary present, eliminates contretemps with traffic, dogs and kibitzers. In fact, it's one of the two exercise aids—the other is the treadmill—that Ken feels is a worthwhile investment. Most devices just don't work in an aerobics program.

Readers of Ken's earlier books know that in principle he's against spending *any* money (except for proper shoes) on aerobics exercise because it simply isn't necessary. He's met too many people who've purchased exercise equipment and then used it for only a short time until their enthusiasm wore off. In the aftermath, they not only felt gypped, but also hostile toward conditioning. Most of the gimmicks that involve pushing or pulling or vibration are designed for muscle toning alone, not cardiovascular conditioning, and if they don't do any harm they certainly don't do any good.

A stationary bicycle, however, can be used very effectively if you observe certain guidelines. Don't use a bike with rowing action handlebars or one that's motorized—the latter results in passive exercise and does nothing to improve the overall condition of your heart and lungs. Do use a bike that has these four basic accessories: an odometer to show how many miles you "travel," an adjustment for varying the resistance of the pedals, a timer, a speedometer.

Since the price of stationary bicycles can range from $30 all the way up to $1,000, you really should do some careful investigating before you make a decision about this purchase.

In general, the cheapest models don't have the basic four accessories and the highest-cost ones have features such as a heart-rate monitor that aren't needed by the average home user. Among the many models in the $60 to $130 range you'll find that a bar for setting pedal resistance, a speedometer and odometer are standard equipment. Here are a few other checkpoints for you to consider as you comparison-shop: comfortable, easy-to-adjust seat; firm, stable frame;

comfortable handlebar position and grip angle; easy-to-adjust pedal resistance and smooth pedal action; adequate chain guards to protect your clothing.

After you've bought your cycle, follow the instructions Ken gives in Chapter 8 for setting the pedal resistance to achieve the necessary pulse rate, and you'll soon be well on your way to a good level of aerobic fitness.

TREADMILL EXERCISERS

People use the phrase "on a treadmill" to suggest a go-nowhere situation. But a treadmill—a platform with a movable belt that allows you to cover "distance" and simulate regular running without real forward motion—can definitely be used to get somewhere in terms of aerobic conditioning. It has advantages similar to the stationary bicycle in that it takes up only a moderate amount of space and can be used by the whole family. These devices are expensive, however—from about $100 to over $3,000.

Models costing a few hundred dollars are propelled by the user's own muscle power. This is fine except that to exercise on them effectively from the aerobic standpoint you must learn to walk or jog without supporting yourself via the side rails provided, and the no-hands technique isn't easy to learn.

Motor-driven treadmills range from $400 to $500 on up. The very expensive treadmills have adjustments and features that are valuable for researchers or physicians but quite unnecessary for the home exerciser. Those suitable for non-professional users have a selection of speeds and sometimes a built-in mechanism for adjusting the amount of incline. (Exercising on an uphill slant earns more aerobic points than running on a level surface, as illustrated in the chart below.)

All treadmill exercise must be accomplished without using your hands. Just select the appropriate age category for walking or running (pages 64-80) and follow it as you would for outdoor conditioning. If you want to use an incline—some treadmills that are not equipped with built-in incline adjustment can simply be raised at the front end with blocks—

the following chart shows you the increased aerobic point values you can earn.

POINT VALUES FOR WALKING/RUNNING ONE MILE
ON A TREADMILL SET AT VARIOUS INCLINES

TREADMILL SPEED (m.p.h.)	MILE/TIME (minutes)	INCLINE (% grade)				
		0%	5%	10%	15%	
10	6:00	6	7	9	— *	
7.5	8:00	5	6	7	10	
6	10:00	4	5	6	7	
5	12:00	3	4	5	6	POINTS
4.14	14:30	2	4	5	6	
3	20:00	1	1½	2½	3	
2.5	25:00	0	1	1½	2	
		0°	3°	6°	9°	
		INCLINE (degrees)				

* This is virtually impossible for anyone but an Olympic athlete.

If your treadmill is motorized and equipped with a speedometer, you can use an alternative means of earning points: Keep the mill flat, set it for one of the speeds in the following chart and stay on it for the number of minutes indicated to earn the number of points shown.

POINTS FOR WALKING/RUNNING ONE MILE
ON A MOTORIZED TREADMILL (No Incline)

TREADMILL SPEED (m.p.h.)	MILE TIME (minutes)	POINTS
10	6:00	6
9¼	6:30	6
8½	7:00	5
8	7:30	5
7½	8:00	5
7	8:30	4
6⅔	9:00	4
6⅓	9:30	4
6	10:00	4
5	12:00	3
4½	13:30	2
4	15:00	1
3½	17:30	1
3	20:00	1

Here and in the previous chapter you've been reading about the "anatomy" of the various indoor and outdoor aerobics programs. Now I'll get more personal and talk about aerobics in terms of its potential effect on the human body—from scalp to sole.

11: Aerobic Fitness from Top to Toes

You MAY THINK I exaggerate when I say that we have had testimonials on the therapeutic value of aerobic exercise in connection with everything from dandruff to toenails and all that goes in between. I'm in earnest. After one of Ken's presentations a man came up to him and said, "You know, I want to report on a strange phenomenon. My toenails had been hurting and feeling as if they were about to fall off. But after I started exercising they were okay again." At the other bodily extremity, some people have told Ken their dandruff improved or disappeared with exercise!

Of course these conditions are probably coincidental and certainly inconsequential compared to the far more serious disabilities that aerobics has benefited. In fact, the spectrum of aerobic therapy is so broad that it makes sense to describe it starting with the head and working down to the feet. It's possible that in doing this I run the risk of making aerobics sound like Dr. Cooper's good-for-what-ails-you patented panacea, but the proven and the potential value of scientifically measured exercise for a wide variety of physical impairments is too great not to share with you what we've learned in the laboratory and what we hear from aerobics practitioners around the country.

A number of people, for example, have written Ken to say that aerobic exercise has helped their migraine headaches. The letter from John Doherty, Jr., of Greenlawn, New York, is typical:

I had migraine attacks that grew progressively worse for 12 years. Almost anything could trigger them. Eventually I was getting 2 or 3 a week and was constantly in "aura"—either going into or recovering from migraine. I was nearly an invalid.

I started jogging and very, very slowly worked up to

30 points. If I overexerted I got a migraine, so that slowed my progress, along with bad weather and sore ankles. But I finally got into good shape—and then I got a migraine that tied me in knots for a week. When that cleared up, I was over the hump and I have only had 2 since, with a few periods of being in the aura.

Actually, I'm still improving gradually with longer stretches between attacks, milder attacks, quicker recoveries and less awareness of aura. I have the same job, same routine, same diet, weigh about 5 pounds less, live in the same place and have the same stresses and strains. I won't speculate on how aerobics cleared this condition up, but jogging is the only new factor in the equation.

Ken can't explain it either, but the personal case histories keep coming. On the subject of headaches and varicose veins, an Ohio woman wrote:

I'm a 40-year-old mother with 6 children ranging from 12 to 21. Although I've had no serious illnesses in my lifetime, I've been bothered since adolescence by severe, chronic headaches lasting 2 or 3 days; in addition, I've had varicose veins since my third pregnancy, 17 years ago, and have had to wear elastic hosiery since that time.

After reading Aerobics, I began the walking program in the Poor category and worked up to 29 points over 4 months. At present I've been free of headaches for 2 months, and my varicose veins have greatly improved, even to the disappearance of discolorations. Today I discarded elastic hose for the first time in 17 years and switched to support stockings. Some discoloration in my ankles still persists, but it's not as noticeable as in the past.

Varicosities are apt to appear in the form of blotchy areas around the ankles. Although they are often a symptom of aging, pregnancy, excess weight and inactivity can also precipitate them. The condition is caused by the lessening of elasticity in the veins; when this happens they tend to sag and allow blood to accumulate or "pool," resulting in discolorations.

Exercise can't be said to cure varicosities because by the time they show up the blood vessels have already deteriorated. But in many instances the varicosities do improve, and I can assure you that if you don't do *something* about them, they'll get even worse. Ken encourages people with this problem to check first with their physicians, then enter one of the aerobics programs and see how they respond. From Ken's standpoint it has to be a kind of trial-and-error approach, but he does feel that regular exercise can induce beneficial changes in many cases.

A lot of people have claimed they've had to get prescription changes in their glasses once they started to exercise because their vision improved. We really don't know enough about these cases to establish a correlation, but Ken has had the experience of working with several patients suffering from open-angle glaucoma, in which pressure builds up inside the eye very gradually until vision blurs—and sometimes fails completely. As he reported in *Aerobics*, exercise proved to be a successful means of lowering tension and pressure in the eyeball.

About teeth, Ken's father, a dentist, says that he can tell when one of his patients is physically fit because of the difference in the color of his gums. The fact is, a person who has used aerobic-type exercise sufficiently to achieve the training effect has an improved blood flow or vascularization that shows up not only in improved gum tissue but in better tissues throughout the body. This is why we can document innumerable cases of reduced blood pressure and lowered cholesterol level commensurate with aerobic exercise.

Your skin, of course, is tissue, and while Ken obviously can't guarantee that exercise does anything in the way of reducing extra chins or tightening up bags under the eyes, he's observed over and over again that a younger look tends to return—there's a rosy blush to the cheek, a definite change in the appearance of the skin tissue. Just a few days ago he came home and told me about a man in his middle forties he'd just evaluated. His skin gave the impression of being so fresh and youthful that he actually seemed to have delayed or reversed the aging process.

If the idea of sweating when you exercise is distasteful to you, give some thought to what it will do for your skin. (Whenever I use the word "sweat," I think of the old saying, "Horses sweat, men perspire and ladies glow." With aerobics, everyone—ladies included—should be prepared to sweat.) Here's a comment from Mrs. Martha Frank of Lake Village, Arkansas, on the effect of sweating on her complexion—Ken also quoted her in *The New Aerobics* on the subject of how she's literally reshaped her legs on the aerobic running program. "When you write your book for women," she said in a recent letter, "tell them that the profuse sweating of my face when I exercise has done something for clearing up my complexion nothing short of what the sauna or Swedish baths are supposed to do. Also I no longer need to use moisture preparations; I suppose because the running has activated my glands and made them work harder. And because my legs are so much firmer, the skin doesn't bruise all the time the way it used to and the little beginnings of broken veins are relieved."

Ken agrees with Mrs. Frank that sweating during exercise has a cleansing effect on the skin, and tends to reduce the need for medications and cosmetics. I personally can chime in on this, too—I have trouble with pimples now and then, but my complexion frequently clears up when I've been exercising.

A few years ago Ken got an intriguing letter from one of the country's leading allergists noting that when she started some of her patients on exercise programs their allergies were attenuated. She felt strongly, she said, that a connection exists between serious allergic conditions and fitness. Ken thinks she may be right—although he doesn't know the reason for it.

Certainly many asthma sufferers have responded remarkably well to exercise. These people are, in general, very sadly deconditioned—since childhood they've been excused from physical education and recreation periods because every time they started exercising they began to wheeze. Yet with carefully supervised, gradually progressive exercise their condition has definitely improved. Annette Racaniello, a sophomore majoring in physical education at Cortland State Teachers' College in New York State, is a young woman who achieved such a high level of fitness while battling allergic bronchial asthma that she won a scholarship from the American Association for Health, Physical Education and Recreation. Do you wonder that this letter from Annette made us feel a bit like proud parents?

"This week I swam about 4½ miles and by the end of the week I will have run about 6 miles. Occasionally I still do have a little trouble with my asthma, but aerobics has helped me more than *any* medication or desensitization treatment. If not for you, I never would have won either of my physical-education scholarships. Your program gave me a unique physical conditioning experience that I wouldn't have believed possible unless I'd tried it."

Asthma puts a strain on the lungs. It makes breathing more difficult and rapid, and this extra burden is comparable to that caused by the coughing that goes with emphysema, tuberculosis and bronchitis. In each of these diseases, aerobic-type exercise—specifically intended to strengthen the lungs and increase their capacity to process air—has been used with good results.

As for heart and blood-vessel disease, if you're not aware by now of aerobics' contribution in terms of prevention, I might as well turn in my typewriter and take a vow of silence. On the rehabilitative side, the account "Mrs. Paxton" gave in Chapter 5 of her return to a normal life is one hundreds of other cardiac patients who've also had aerobic therapy could tell.

Exercise promotes reduced stress and tension and this is a factor not only in lowering blood pressure but also in counteracting the hyperacidity that attacks the stomach lining and contributes to ulcers. Ken cited one medical article on this antiulcergenic effect when his first book was published in 1968 and since then several more documentary studies have come out substantiating this effect.

In diabetes, where the body's ability to assimilate sugar is impaired, adult patients in particular have combined physical conditioning with special diets and weight-loss programs to cut down on the amount of insulin they need to take. It has been shown recently that conditioned diabetics seem to be more responsive to insulin and therefore to require less of it.

Since I covered the uses of exercise in connection with menstruation, pregnancy and menopause in Chapter 3, and since aerobics is discussed in connection with reducing diets and aging in Chapters 12 and 13, I won't go into its therapeutic value in these areas here. Two problems I do want to mention, though, are constipation and—an especially sensitive concern for women—urinary control.

As Ken puts it, "There's no such thing as a constipated jogger." Exercise stimulates the gastrointestinal muscles and as a result activates the bowels. It's just as effective as a laxative. Regular elimination deriving from regular exercise is something you can count on.

Incontinence or absence of urinary control isn't talked about very often for obvious reasons. Wetting your pants when you cough or laugh or sneeze is annoying, uncomfortable and downright embarrassing. Yet it's a complaint common to our sex, one that frequently crops up after pregnancy. It's caused by a cystocele—a weakness in the bladder walls—and can be corrected by surgery, or sometimes by simply concentrating on controlling the sphincter. This valve-like muscle has the function of closing bodily channels and you can contract the one in the vaginal area voluntarily. Many women have been surprised to find that an incontinence problem improved or disappeared once they started an exercise program. Ken is sure this happens because they unconsciously concentrate on keeping the sphincter closed for the 10, 15 or 20 minutes they're exercising. Theoretically, anyone who *consciously* made an effort to reinforce the sphincter muscle by contracting and releasing it during exercise could also achieve this control.

It may seem contradictory to claim that with exercise you'll feel less tired and sleep better, but it's true. Ken's research with the manned orbiting laboratory program and other studies he conducted, as well as countless "unofficial" reports from exercisers, verify this. Because multiple systems of your body—cardiovascular, pulmonary, digestive, muscular—are responsive to the aerobic training effect, each one of them works more efficiently and effortlessly, keeping energy in reserve, sparing you fatigue and making you more alert. Then, when you get into your bed at night, you're relaxed. The fatigue you do feel is the good, healthy kind that lets you drop off quickly and actually get more rest out of fewer hours' sleep. Ken and I have yet to meet an aerobics exerciser who has a major problem with insomnia.

With this newfound capacity for relaxing, the simple nervous system actually shows some physiological changes. The exercised person becomes less depressed, less hypochondriacal. It's even been documented that such things as absenteeism from work and accidents tend to decrease and productivity to increase.

Peace of mind is part of what helps people sleep well and that usually means a head clear of anxiety. One of Ken's Air Force studies on the "apprehension response" illustrates how regular exercisers don't get as keyed-up or excited. In the beginning stages of testing deconditioned men, he found that the subjects' hearts would begin to race in anticipation of the exercise. Just thinking about the trial that lay ahead would throw a man into a panic that his heart rate reflected. It would go up to 120 or so before he even started to run. Yet once that same man was trained and physically conditioned, he could face the threat of exercise with a remarkably decreased apprehension response. His heart rate rarely exceeded 65 or 70 prior to the run. Also he seemed less inclined to worry or fret so much about the normal stresses of life.

I've left until last an area of aerobic fitness I don't know how to label—whether to call it spiritual or psychological or emotional. An experience Ken had during an appearance on a call-in program on radio may give you an idea of what I'm driving at. A young mother telephoned and told him she was 29 years old and ran 2 miles 4 or

5 times a week, taking her 2 children to the track with her. "There are things about this conditioning program you didn't mention in your book," she said. "I mean intangibles like the new attitude I bring to my children and to the relationship with my husband. I know you can't document these things by putting a blood-pressure cuff on the arm or measuring oxygen consumption, but they're real and they're important to the quality of our lives."

Perhaps the word I'm searching for is "compatibility." There aren't many couples, I suppose, who don't have an argument now and then. Ken thinks nothing's better for clearing the air than a good hard workout. If we have harsh words, likely as not he'll say, "I'm going out and run." It gives us both a chance to cool off and when he comes back we're both ready to smooth things out.

For my part, exercise in general has helped me handle irritability better, to try harder to live up to a passage from I Corinthians, Chapter XIII, that means a great deal to me personally:

"Love is slow to lose patience. It looks for a way of being constructive. It is not possessive. It is neither anxious to impress, nor does it cherish inflated ideas of its own importance. Love has good manners and does not pursue selfish advantage. It is not touchy. It does not keep account of evil, nor gloat over the wickedness of other people. On the contrary, it is glad with all good men when truth prevails. Love knows no limits to its endurance, no end to its trust, no fading of its hope. It can outlast anything. It is, in fact, the only thing that still stands when all else has fallen."

12: A Loving Approach to Diet and Aerobics

WHOEVER YOU ARE, you've got something great going for you: Being you.

This may seem an odd beginning to a discussion of diet and exercise. But having given a lot of thought to the best way to approach my own goals, I've concluded that a positive attitude is essential. Nothing else will get you started and keep you going. It does me no good at all to beat on myself, to chastise and castigate myself for not always doing what I think I ought to do. I have to like myself, basically, and know my assets and take a compassionate attitude toward my weaknesses if I want to make any progress. (I'd be appalled if anyone reading this imagined for one moment that I'm not weak, that exercising regularly and keeping my weight down aren't hard for me, that I don't have to make a fresh start over and over again.)

For one thing, I'm a foodoholic. If you don't happen to live to eat, as I do, you may find that particular compulsion hard to understand. If you're someone who is deaf to the siren call of a dish of peanuts, who can look with dispassionate eyes on a rich dessert, you probably feel impatient with those of us who are so susceptible to snacking and general overeating. You'd be hard put to imagine what a challenge it is to have to apply cease-and-desist discipline to food and to meet that challenge day and night, week in and week out.

A good way to understand, respect and cope with your own hangups, I've found, is to compare them with other people's. For example, nonsmokers—like me—find it hard to appreciate how poignant a smoker's yearning for tobacco is. But by comparing it to my own food craving, I *can* appreciate the effort that goes into restraint. Quiet, reflective types can't understand the need of a voluble person—like me—to run on endlessly, while I'm equally dismayed by even a companionable silence. Sedentary people find the prospect of exercise disagreeable. Active people see nothing funny in the famous remark, "Whenever I feel the need to exercise I lie down until it passes." As a teetotaler, I can't comprehend the pleasure many men and women get from having a few cocktails, and even social drinkers are at a loss to understand the cruel obsession that drives others to addictive drinking and alcoholism.

When you stop to think about it, most of us have excesses of one kind or another, along with soft spots in our willpower. What costs one woman next to nothing in terms of self-control, another woman pays a high price for. The point is, accept yourself as you are. Try approaching goals that involve a change from comfortable and accustomed routine with good will, compassion, a sense of humor and a readiness to keep trying. If you tell yourself sternly, "I've got to do this and I'm rotten if I don't," you're giving yourself a hind-start. I'm not encouraging you to make excuses for lapses, just to be realistic about your expectations.

Acknowledge your assets. Take credit for all the good things you are and do, *even though they come naturally.* Don't devalue an accomplishment or an asset simply because you didn't struggle and suffer for it. Appreciate yourself sincerely. You aren't risking arrogance or heading for a fall if you allow yourself some honest pride, whether it's in your beautifully kept wardrobe or your meticulously swept house.

Admit a deficit. If honest self-esteem comes hard, honest self-criticism is even harder. Americans seem particularly given to euphemisms, to calling a spade an entrenching tool. An obese person is chubby, plump, heavyset, well-endowed, big, hefty—never (shhhhhh!) fat. A person who drinks to the point of alcoholism tipples, overindulges, likes the sauce, drowns his sorrows—a sot he's not. We're not sick, we're ill, indisposed, ailing, under the weather. And on and on. No wonder Roget got a thesaurus out of it. Yet one of

Ken's most successful patients was a high-level airline executive whose wife one day took a straight, level look at him (and probably a deep breath) and said, "Hon, you're getting old and you're getting fat."

And her husband took it like a man. He said, "Yes, I guess you're right." Today, 3 years and a lot of diet and exercise later, he's incalculably more youthful in appearance, outlook and vitality. He may not be a young man, but he's a new man. I often wonder what the result would have been if his wife had said, "Hon, you're getting some very distinguished gray hair and you certainly look like a substantial citizen."

The people who direct the Alcoholics Anonymous program and most other experts on this disease can't begin to help the compulsive drinker until he has admitted that he can't control his drinking. Psychiatrists can't deal with their patients' destructive angers until the troubled one can say, "I'm angry." You can't do one thing about excess weight or a deconditioned body till you take off your rose-colored glasses.

Once you've admitted to this particular problem, a combination of diet and exercise can be incredibly effective in reducing your weight and firming your body tissue at the same time—much more so than either a weight-loss plan or aerobics by itself. As a rather extreme, and highly convincing, example of how this acceptance works, I'd like to tell you about my sister Alice.

Alice is a genuinely pretty woman in her early forties, with a special softness and femininity that I don't have. She's 5'5" tall and has velvety skin, glossy hair, beautifully shaped nose and hands, a lovely singing voice—and until quite recently she weighed 242 pounds.

If your first reaction was a gasp, your second was probably, "Thank goodness my problem isn't *that* bad." Ah, but losing 8 pounds can be harder than losing 80. If you've got a reasonable amount of weight to lose, you're apt to think, "I can take care of that any time" and then go right on procrastinating indefinitely.

Alice's confrontation with herself came at a family wedding, when Ken noticed a drastic worsening of the varicose veins in her legs. (Like the rest of our relatives, he'd avoided bringing up her obesity because he knew she was so painfully sensitive about it. But now the varicosity was so bad that veins in one leg were "weeping." She had a condition called pitting edema, meaning the swelling is so serious it retains the mark of a thumbprint for an hour or more.)

"Alice," Ken asked, "*what* do you weigh?"

"I don't know."

"Alice, you're going to lose that leg and possibly your life if you don't face up to what you are. Go on in and weigh yourself." He was so furious and she was so frightened, I was sure that, if nothing else, this was the end of our friendly family relationship.

"Ken, I just ate," she pleaded.

"Alice, *go in and weigh*."

Two forty-two. Later she admitted she hadn't weighed under 200 pounds in 10 years—and firmly believed she never would.

"I want you to go home and put a sign with 'two forty-two' on it everywhere you look—your walls, your refrigerator, your scale," Ken told her. "But before you do that, you're going to have to go to the hospital because you're on the borderline of losing that leg."

Alice went to the hospital the next morning and stayed one month. During that time, between draining fluid and the hospital diet, she lost 22 pounds and the doctors were able to inject her varicosities. They found a tiny incidence of a thyroid condition, but not enough to account for the excessive weight.

All through her hospital stay, Alice was one depressed woman. The limited diet frustrated her so much that she'd beg her husband to smuggle in extra food. When my mother visited her she'd hide her head under the covers and cry. My father drove her mad because—having just successfully accomplished a weight loss to combat a medical problem—he knew how to *preach*. He'd tell the dieticians they were putting three times too much food on her trays.

After she left the hospital, Alice found the battle had barely been engaged. The doctor advised her to eat evening meals at my parents' house because Mother works in a hospital kitchen preparing dietetic meals and knew how to give her nourishing menus that would help her take off weight. Meantime, Ken set up an individual aerobics program for her—stationary cycling in the morning and walking in the evening—and asked her to keep daily records of her weight and report to him on her progress every week.

Alice continued to have a defeatist attitude about herself. The distance she had to travel seemed so endless. Like all of us, she'd find excuses. My father is on an aerobics program too, and when he'd urge her to come out walking with him after dinner she'd complain about her sore feet and blisters. She'd tell Ken how impractical it all was. But everyone kept after her. (There are times when we *do* need someone to nag and hound us.)

And slowly the tide of the battle began to turn. One day Alice glanced down at her legs and they looked so different she couldn't believe it. She tried on the dress she'd been wearing when Ken first made her weigh herself and it literally swallowed her. She discovered she'd lost 4 inches on her upper arms alone. And when her 23-year-old daughter and her husband came to visit her, they couldn't keep up with her on a mile-and-a-half walk.

So far, Alice has lost about 55 pounds. She still has a long way to go before she reaches her goal. Like the Alcoholics Anonymous participants, she needs constant encouragement and support. But the weight loss she has accomplished with diet and exercise to date has also resulted in intangible gains that will help her go the rest of the way: she has a brand-new sense of self-respect and self-confidence.

Primarily, she has educated herself to a whole new way of life. She has learned to prepare her own dietetic meals in her own home, without being tempted to cheat. She cycles and walks every day. She isn't threatened or demoralized by those not-so-well-meaning people who say, "You're looking awfully tired, I hope it isn't too much for you," or "I know you're trying to lose weight, but your face doesn't seem as sweet and pretty as it did before." (Alice knows that her pretty face drew all the attention because there wasn't much to compliment about the rest of her.)

I'm thoroughly convinced that the heart of Alice's problem was that *she could not admit to herself what she had become,* and that remission from it began when *she acknowledged the problem.*

One last word on my sister. My parents have a clock with a cheerful little boy and girl who swing in and out of doorways when it chimes. Alice used to hate it. "Look at that pair," she'd say. "They look so happy. I can't understand people who look as if they're happy all the time." Now Alice is beginning to understand—and time, once the thief and the enemy, is now her ally.

AEROBICS COMBINED WITH A REDUCING PLAN

It's well worth repeating that a reduced-calorie diet and regular exercise are a natural combination since the goals of each are parallel and they both call for a daily effort and perseverance that don't come easily. To review the facts about diet and exercise:

With exercise alone, you won't lose weight *rapidly* though you'll lose inches. However, it's almost inevitable that you lose some weight if you exercise consistently over a long period of time.

Example: If you walk a mile in 20 minutes or run a mile in 8 minutes, you burn up 75-100 calories. Say you run a mile and a half daily 5 times a week for a total of 750 calories burned. You need to burn approximately 3,300 calories to lose a pound, so you could expect to lose a pound a month if you exercised regularly without changing your eating habits at all. If you continued to exercise, you'd lose 6 pounds in 6 months or 12 pounds a year. Not spectacular, but the cumulative effect can work to your advantage.

By combining an aerobics program of moderate intensity —jogging, cycling, swimming, stationary running—with a reduced-calorie diet, you can anticipate losing weight at a much speedier rate, and you lose fat tissue only—without depleting muscle mass. (On a purely fasting program of water and vitamin pills, you would lose half fat and half muscle and wind up with unattractive, sagging tissues.) The combination of a well-balanced, reduced-calorie menu plan and exercise results in lean firm tissues all over, and they're the bikini type, not the musclebound kind.

Example: Eliminate 500 calories a day from your usual intake and burn up another 750 calories by exercising 5 days a week. With this formula, you could look for a weekly weight loss of at least 1¼ pounds for a minimum of 5 pounds a month (for the average person, doctors feel a loss of 1 to 2 pounds a week is safest).

It's true that light exercise—walking a mile in 20 minutes, for example—may have the effect of stimulating your appetite, and also that a single soft drink afterward can restore the 100 calories you've just burned up. You have to be wary of this.

On the other hand, vigorous exercise tends to depress the appetite (it shunts blood away from the stomach, decreasing the desire for food), which is why Ken urges people to exercise just before a meal.

You can use exercise to burn up specific caloric amounts by referring to Ken's special charts in the Appendix, pages 156-9. He has matched the caloric values of typical servings of about a hundred popular foods and beverages with the exact amount of aerobic exercise you need to perform to work them off. While it may be discouraging to you to know, for example, that you have to walk 1½ miles in 30 minutes, run a mile in 8 minutes, or cycle 3 miles in 12 minutes to burn up the 120 calories in a single 1-ounce piece of chocolate fudge, it may also do wonders for your willpower.

However you look at it, these charts can be an invaluable tool in helping you plan either compensatory exercise or explicit goals for losing weight via aerobics.

Changing your metabolic pattern is possible when you combine diet with exercise. That is, Ken has supervised a number of cases in which the individual has reduced his weight to the ideal level, and then has resumed his pre-diet eating habits without putting on weight. In every instance, the key factor was regular, continuing exercise.

If you're fat, it's pretty demoralizing to contemplate the idea of being on a diet the rest of your life, and this is what many obese people expect, having experienced a vicious gain-and-lose, gain-and-lose cycle in the past. But if you know there are men and women who lose weight and go back to almost the same eating pattern they were on formerly *without* gaining, the picture is much brighter. The ordeal of dieting becomes temporary, transient and feasible. With exercise as the continuing factor, keeping in shape once you've reached your weight goal isn't nearly as hard as *getting* in shape.

I don't mean to raise hopes falsely. The fat man or woman does have an above-average capacity for storing fat, combined with reduced metabolic action. But many who change from an obese state to a lean state using a diet-exercise plan find they can eat without restriction and not gain because their metabolism has changed.

Although he doesn't regard them as documentary, Ken has recorded several examples of this phenomenon. One is my father. Ken put him on a 1,000-calorie diet combined with a walking program and he dropped from 198 to 156 pounds in 3 months; his triglyceride level went down from an astronomical figure to normal and even his blood pressure was lowered. Dad had lunch with us recently and we were astonished by the amount of starchy food he ate. But he doesn't worry about gaining weight any more. He's still exercising, and he just doesn't metabolize food the way he did before.

Another man, a commercial airlines pilot, 5'8", started out weighing 190 pounds. Ken put him on a walking-running program and a 1,000-calories-a-day reducing diet. He got stuck at 170 pounds and couldn't seem to get any lower —on 1,000 calories he was almost gaining weight even though he was walking 2 or 3 miles a day. He got things moving again by dropping down to about 500 calories daily for about 10 days. When he finally leveled off at 155 pounds, he also stabilized there because his metabolism had changed, and because he continued exercising.

A woman patient had a similar pattern in reducing from 135 to 120 pounds. At a certain point she plateaued, just like the pilot. She limited her food intake to a liquid nutritional supplement for 4 days, started losing again, made her ideal weight and maintained it without any further need for dieting. She continued the walking/running program Ken prescribed for her and at the age of 48 she has what he calls a "fantastic" figure.

THE REDUCING DIET ITSELF

If one subject is more abused in this country than exercise, it's diet. So many false claims are made and, even worse, believed! And yet, as with exercise, there just isn't any easy way to diet and lose weight—no candy, no magic combination of foods, no seven-day-wonder plans, no machines, gadgets, belts or special wearing apparel can substitute for keeping track of your caloric intake faithfully and limiting it judiciously.

Since lists of the specific groups that should be represented in your diet every day can be found in many cookbooks, in government pamphlets, in library books and in free folders distributed by national health associations and by numerous companies, I won't restate them here. Just bear in mind the two cardinal rules for a reducing diet: it must contain all the necessary daily nutrients required by your body, with emphasis on lean meats, fish, poultry, fresh vegetables and low-saturated fats; it should, like your exercise program, have your doctor's approval.

Protecting your health is a way of bettering your chances to be around that much longer to love and be loved. *Now* you see where I got the title for this chapter.

13: Too Young or Too Old? Hardly Ever!

THE NATURAL AFFINITY between older people and the young has been observed often—the mutual confidence, affection and patience that's invariably seen in the relationship between grandparents and their grandchildren, and for that matter between oldsters and youngsters who aren't related at all. I bring this up because I sometimes suspect that one thing that makes a bridge between generations widely separated in years is the fact that they experience a common denial—they're told repeatedly, "It's too soon" or "It's too late," "You're too young" or "You're too old."

In some cases, the time may *be* wrong, or gone, for certain experiences or activities. But that's rarely true of aerobic exercise. You need it when you're reasonably young to form the habit, and to reinforce your health when your body's natural fitness peaks in the teens. You need it in your mature years to help make them as vital and free of inhibiting physical ailments as humanly possible.

On the subject of youth and exercise, I want to mention at the very outset how much I admire the work being done via the "Special Olympics" for retarded children, an event including running, swimming and other active sports held in several regions of the United States and Canada each summer. It's sponsored by the Joseph P. Kennedy, Jr., Foundation and it's designed to demonstrate the need—and value—of physical-fitness training for retarded youngsters from 8 to 18 years old. Studies on mentally retarded children have shown that participation in vigorous physical exercise can result in a marked improvement in these children's classroom work habits, and increase their general performance level and ability to enter into community life.

Many people harbor the illusion that children "just

naturally" get enough exercise without making a conscious effort. How wrong they are. As an example, unfortunately one of many, of the typical unfitness of American youngsters, here are the results of the 12-minute aerobics running test (run as far as you can in 12 minutes) administered to young girls at a Jacksonville, Florida, junior high school. In this study of 502 participants between 12 and 15 years old, conducted by Patricia Ann Hielscher, 324 fell into the Very Poor category—they were unable to cover a mile. Another 148 were Poor, unable to cover more than 1.14 mile; only 28 were Fair, able to cover between 1.15 and 1.34 mile; just 2 were Good, able to cover 1.35 to 1.64 mile. *None* qualified for the Excellent conditioning category, over 1.65 mile. I cite these disturbing figures not as an indictment of one particular school in Florida, but of the physical-education programs in a majority of schools throughout the country.

Nor do I feel the full responsibility for generating interest in exercise should fall on the public schools. Physical fitness, like charity, begins at home. My answer to mothers who ask, "But how can I get my children to exercise?" is very simple: "Set the example." Children learn by watching their parents.

Now if you just tell your child, "Get out there and run some laps," you're bound to get resistance. Take my own 5-year-old daughter. When I go out to exercise in our back-yard, I don't say, "Come on out and join me, Berkley." But seeing me, she'll usually volunteer, "Mommie, I want to jog with you."

As a mother myself, I can sympathize with the conflict parents may feel—when you love someone you want to *do* for them, make their life as convenient as possible. Yet in the case of exercise, you're doing them an injustice if you excuse them from it or try to spare them the effort. One instance of this—my pet peeve—is driving kids to so many of their appointments. At the very least, they can be encouraged to walk on errands or ride their bicycles.

I *do* feel we have a long way to go in implementing good conditioning programs in junior high and high schools.

People frequently ask Ken when a child should start a conditioning program, and if sex or age makes a difference. He did a study on boys and girls, about equally divided, between the ages of 6 and 12 that was designed to measure their oxygen consumption during field tests. Up to roughly 10 years of age, he found no marked contrast between the sexes in their aerobic capacity based on maximum oxygen consumption. As a result, when the Physical Fitness Committee of the American College of Pediatrics asked him for specific instructions on aerobic-type conditioning programs for schools' physical-fitness programs, he recommended no regimentation up to about age 10. Ken feels that until that time, youngsters are normally quite active on their own and if you start trying to *make* them do something on a disciplined basis, it tends to discourage them and interfere with their spontaneous enjoyment.

However, once they're into the fifth and sixth grades, or ages 11 or 12, he thinks it's time to introduce some reasonable, semiformal fitness program—one interesting and varied enough to stave off boredom. It's exactly then when the aerobic "equalness" begins to change—the boys continue to improve in their endurance and the girls to level off and stabilize. So you should be challenging one sex and supporting the other.

Unless there's reinforcement at that point, the sad consequences are evident later on. Testimony to this fact is a famous study made by William F. Enos and reported in the *Journal of the American Medical Association,* July 18, 1953. He reported that among 200 American servicemen with an average age of 22.1 years who were killed in Korea, 77.3 percent already had some gross evidence of coronary arteriosclerosis (hardening of the arteries). That statistic alone is enough to convince me that if we want to use public-school conditioning programs as part of the means of preventing heart disease and of changing national health habits, they must begin early—in junior high or before.

I'd hate to give you the impression that schools are ignoring the significance of statistics like these. Far from it. One program that Ken likes to mention—it's duplicated in a number of schools—was initiated at Orange View Junior High School in Anaheim, California, in September 1968. The physical education department decided to award grades based on the distance boys could run in 12 minutes (currently versions of this program are being used in various parts of the country with girls, too). The teachers announced to parents that the boys, about 13½ years old, would not earn an A in P.E. at the end of the school year unless they could run 1.75 miles in less than 12 minutes. A B grade called for running 1.50 miles; a C, 1.25 miles; a D, one mile, and under a mile rated F.

At first the parents objected when they heard their children would be graded this way, but they agreed to accept the program on a trial basis. The modus operandi was for the boys to run up to a mile or a mile and a half before every P.E. class and then go on to the usual sports and activities. Just compare these figures for an idea of what aerobic training did for 367 youngsters: when they were first tested, only 4 percent made A and 29 percent B; by June, the conditioning had worked so well that 37.7 percent earned A and 52.2 percent B.

(I feel compelled to add a few words here of praise and sorrow regarding the Golden State. Until recently physical education was mandatory in its school systems; as a result, California youngsters were so far physically superior to kids from other sections of the country that Ken could spot them immediately when they came into Lackland Air Force Base. Now, however, they may not be so wonderfully recognizable.)

As for girls' response to aerobic training in their P.E. classes, a study conducted by Welta Burris, a dynamic young instructor at Lee High School in San Antonio, gives a good picture. In January 1969, she tested 96 girls of about 14½, whose average weight was 119 pounds, average height, about 5'4". At the beginning of the semester, only 26.1 percent could run further than 1.15 miles in 12 minutes. For the next 5 weeks, 4 times a week, she simply had the girls run continuously for 5 minutes, building up to 8 minutes. When she tested them again, the percentage of those who could do more than 1.15 miles in 12 minutes jumped from 26.1 to 64.8. The point is, a great deal can be accomplished very easily in very little time.

Imaginative goals are great for motivating kids. I particularly liked a gambit used at the junior high school in North Mankato, Minnesota. One class competed against another to see which group of students could be first to log enough miles-run to equal the distance between their town and various cities in Minnesota. The youngsters enjoyed the challenge so much they actually stayed around after school hours and used their free periods to run and build up the miles needed for their class to win the race.

Not long ago, one of the Des Moines newspapers reported on a study of 300 local high school students in which they were asked, "Are you getting enough exercise?" The interviewers got a negative answer from 87 percent of these teen-agers. They said they weren't getting enough exercise at school or at home. And one of them made a very astute observation. He said, "I look at my mom and dad right now and I see a very low level of fitness. They exercised a whole lot more when they were my age than I'm exercising. What am *I* going to look like when I'm *their* age?"

If anyone reading this is worrying about the size and value of the legacy they'll be able to leave their children, I suggest that the focus be physical rather than financial. When you invest a concern for fitness in your heirs, together with a determination to earn it, your gift is measureless, priceless—and tax-free.

Many young adults are becoming aware that they don't have the physical exertions present in their lives that their parents did. Consider today's young, topflight executives whose minds have been given the best schooling and professional training—yet at age 35 and younger, heart disease is knocking them out. Cardiovascular disease alone accounts for 31 percent of all deaths of men and women between ages 35 and 44. What difference do high salaries, honors, prestige and charisma make if you are physically depleted or incapacitated? If you're saving money for your golden retirement years, why spend them in a wheelchair going to bed at seven p.m. with a glass of warm milk?

The majority of our mail comes from middle-aged housewives and the elderly—the women whose children have moved away. For them, the traditional goals have already been accomplished: love, marriage, children, perhaps grandchildren. They look more favorably on exercise because they realize they *don't* have youth going for them and that they're going to have to put forth some extra effort. When your body starts to age, you lose a degree of confidence. At first it's all a blossoming process, but once you get past 35, you realize that to keep any bloom on your body you're going to have to work at it. The shine is not as bright unless you do something to maintain it. You feel something slipping at this point.

Life tends to make a full circle. You go from complete dependency back to complete dependency unless you prepare yourself. With the national population in general, and women in particular, living many years longer, the problem of aging has become the problem of how to remain productive and useful. I think there can be no question that exercise for the premenopausal woman is a must. Apart from the physiological benefits, it's essential psychologically for her to follow the traditional accomplishments with something else, and what better than a program to keep her body fit and ready for all the life that's still ahead? Obviously, I'm not recommending that anyone deliberately wait till age 40 or so to begin conditioning, but if you *have* delayed, please don't waste another minute.

About once a year, Ken and I get down to McAllen, Texas, a town whose balmy winter climate attracts retirement-age people from all over the country. Frankly, some older people depress me because they remind me of how fast my own life is slipping away. But not those I saw in McAllen. They were having more fun! They walked, bicycled, played in shuffleboard tournaments. The key factor in their lives was *doing* something. You have to keep active or you might as well be dead. In my opinion, if you don't have any more mountains to climb, any more goals to achieve, you *are* dead. You're just eating and breathing and existing and drifting and missing the joy of living that can be yours at any age.

At any age? Yes indeed. Ken has shown that people of 70 years and much older can achieve an aerobic training response. And listen to this letter excerpt I quote in all my presentations:

> *Dear Dr. Cooper:*
>
> *I want to take this opportunity to thank you for the aerobics conditioning program. I have followed it faithfully for 9 months. During the past 6 months, I have been averaging at least 30 points a week entirely by walking. I sleep better, feel better and have gone through the winter without any medical problems for the first time, and I am eagerly awaiting my ninety-fourth birthday.*

Ken gets so many letters from members of the Seniors Track Club—some in their sixties and up—who love to send him the results of races in which they've outperformed younger people. I personally am fascinated by the tri-wheeler clubs that are cropping up—this kind of cycle seems to be a favorite among older people—and I treasure a letter we received from Miss Rose M. Coventry of Boise, Idaho:

> *Because I have had a lack of muscle coordination from birth, I was unable to learn to ride a regular bicycle. At age 55, I purchased a 3-gear adult tri-wheeler. Since I have been riding, I have improved in health. Even my friends tell me how much better I look. I am not so nervous, my appetite is keener, and the calf of my right leg, which had become stiff after removal of the head of the fibula, is now as flexible as the other calf. . . . Have you considered working out a chart tri-wheel riders might use? I had in mind that senior citizens in housing projects might enjoy earning aerobic points on a tri-wheeler if it were community property and they could take turns.*

(Ken encourages people over 60 to use a tri-wheeler in the basic aerobics cycling program; the chart on time goals, points and distances appears on page 81.)

In earlier chapters, I've discussed the specific physical benefits of aerobic exercise to the older woman in terms of recovering from surgical procedures, menopause, reversing the effect of aging and so on. One last thought. If you have a friend or relative in a nursing home who isn't getting exercise voluntarily or through an established program in the home, consider taking it upon yourself to urge him or her to do so. Merely walking daily can diminish the symptoms that go with advanced years and a sedentary life. Purposeful conditioning activity can improve sleep, tone muscles, eliminate incontinence, decrease susceptibility to bone fracture and brighten mental outlook and awareness.

As for the person who looks back from your mirror—it's never too late. And it's later than you think.

14: Getting Aerobics Together—with Your Family, Your Man, Your Friends

"My family enjoys exercise as much as I do," Mrs. Emma Childers, a 35-year-old Whittier, California, mother wrote in a letter to Ken. "On weekends we all go to the track and my husband flies kites or plays football and baseball with our 10-year-old son while I run. Some of my little daughter's pleasantest hours have been spent playing in the sand in the long-jump pit. Even though our boy doesn't do much long-distance running (he fancies himself a sprinter), he is in excellent condition and can easily go out and crank off 3 or 4 miles if he wants to. He's had some good exposure to track and field events and to athletes that many other children have never had and recently won 5 out of 6 possible gold medals at the local Cub Scout Olympics. In addition, my 70-year-old father-in-law is on a running program since reading your book and does a mile a day faithfully, *up* and down hill."

Not incidentally, as a result of Mrs. Childers' taking up aerobic exercise—stationary running at first, and then running on a track—she became interested in competitive running. Now she routinely places third or fourth in cross-country events with younger women and has become one of the few American women to complete a classic, 26-mile marathon, placing 169th in a field of 288 starters.

"The marvelous thing is the way running makes you feel physically," she says. "I hear many women complain about feeling tired. I rarely feel physically fatigued. I make all my own bread, sew most of my own and my daughter's clothes, do the cooking, washing, chauffeuring, yard work, painting and anything else that comes up. I'm not bragging (or griping). The point I'm trying to make is that I've noticed all the women I know who run seem to have a high energy rate.

"One of the nicest bonuses is that people compliment you on your figure. Not a week goes by that my husband hasn't thanked me for keeping my figure in shape. Since I'm tall and thin, I've always had shapeless legs, but now my husband tells me how good-looking and filled out they've become. Many women ask me if I'm wearing a girdle (almost never) because my 'bottom is so firm.'

"Before I read *Aerobics,* I didn't know what a pulse rate was or the significance of it. Now I'm quite a boaster about my low pulse rate. Recently I had to have a physical and after listening to my heart the doctor had me run in place for a minute. When I was through he listened to my heart again and then told the nurse in mock seriousness, 'I don't think we can sign her form or allow her to run anymore —her heart rate went from 52 all the way up to 60.' When I compare this to my friends whose resting heart rates are 95, I can't help feeling superior."

Obviously, everyone in this family profits on many levels from Mrs. Childers' love of exercise, and her letter should be reassuring to any woman who fears that her conditioning program will take time away from her family. The way around that, clearly, is to exercise *as* a family.

In San Antonio, during the seasons when we still had daylight after dinner, it was so encouraging to Ken and me to drive over to the high school track and see whole families exercising. The father would be running or jogging around the course and maybe the mother would be walking fast and the kids would be going about half a lap and then sprinting out to the middle of the field to kick a ball. Everyone would be going at their own pace, doing their own thing.

If there's a track in your neighborhood, I urge you to exploit it just as you would a park or recreation area. Take your children over regularly—you can push your baby in his stroller for a couple of laps and keep an eye on the older ones at the same time.

Family exercise, by the way, can be critically important

in some instances. In the last 10 years or so, doctors have recognized the value of supervised exercise for asthmatic patients, and Ken found in working with asthmatic children that the only way he could get them into an exercise program successfully was to encourage the whole family to participate. These youngsters were apprehensive of doing anything on their own. They had no reserve capacity at all, so they were obliged to start from scratch in their walking and eventual running programs. The magic trick was to get the mother to go out with these boys and girls and walk with them. This really had a positive effect on the kids.

Asthmatic or not, it's obvious that children who see their parents exercising are subtly nudged toward getting into it themselves. However, as far as daily activities and controlling the routine of the family are concerned, the mother is probably more important than the father. Ken has emphasized in his lectures and presentations that if we want to start practicing effective preventive medicine in this country in the area of coronary disease, education on food and fitness has to begin in junior high school. Here again, the mother rather than the father is in the position of having the most contact with their children. Her own attitude toward conditioning, the meals she serves, the things she teaches her children about preparing foods and selecting ones that are low in various types of fats and provide correct nutritional balance—all this adds up to a priceless contribution in education and motivation.

THE PLEASURE—AND IMPORTANCE—OF HIS COMPANY

Women's influence on the men in their lives is talked and written about often enough, but I wonder how many actually take advantage of that very real and wonderful opportunity to have a positive effect.

A woman is pretty much responsible for even the morale and mood in the house. If she's poor in spirit when her husband gets home, it's not going to take long for her to infect him. If she's in a good humor, the couple is likely to have a pleasant evening.

As for a man's physical condition and his participation in a conditioning program, his wife's attitude can make all the difference in the world. That's not just my personal opinion. In a study made by the U.S. Public Health Service, the men whose wives encouraged them or participated with them in their exercise had a dropout rate of only 20 percent. For those whose wives had a negative attitude, the dropout rate was over 60 percent!

I know a lawyer's wife whose whole family laughed at her determination to do aerobic exercise. She'd get their breakfast ready and then go out to a vacant lot across the street and run laps. Then when the benefits started to show up, they stopped laughing so much. She never said a word to them, nothing to turn them off—just persisted—and finally her husband began to join her. Her example was worth a thousand nagging words. We also know a group of women in the South who tried like mad to get their husbands active in exercise—talked it up, pleaded and prodded—because these men were just going along getting older and fatter The wives were seriously concerned about the men's very lives, they'd become so coronary-prone. The women got nowhere so they started their own jogging program. They accomplished so much in terms of weight loss and improving their figures that eventually their husbands were literally embarrassed into exercising, too.

Of course, the ideal time for men and women to start programming fitness into their lives is in the late teens and early twenties, the years when the tendency to gain begins. One of the many Air Force studies Ken made shows this upswing graphically. During an 11-year period, from age 19 to 29, the average airman would gain 11 pounds. If he came into the service at 19 weighing 159 pounds, he weighed 170 at 29. He didn't gain a pound a year, he'd put on 6 pounds in a 2- to 3-year period, roughly between ages 22 and 25. This is significant because the average marriage age for American men is 22.8 years. So you see what a key influence a young wife can be in this critical time span, especially since "settling down" into marriage usually means less concentration on fitness activity—

and for the woman herself, the extra physical burden of childbearing.

So far, I've been dwelling on the woman's role in motivating a man to exercise. But once you arouse his interest, you've got an opportunity for so much fun and gratification in exercising together. I like the way Marilyn Van Derbur, former Miss America, now television personality, corporate consultant and a good friend, puts it:

"For 7 years, my husband and I have been running 2 to 3 miles several times a week. It's exciting and exhilarating. We've watched the sun come up so many mornings; we've felt the hot sun on our faces; the crisp fall air in our lungs; the snow crunching under our running shoes. It has become one of the things we most enjoy doing together.

"Our exercise program has brought us, we believe, more vitality, less nervous tension, better health, a common interest and, not incidentally, it contributed to a perfectly delightful birth experience—a baby girl brought into the world quickly and without the dulling effects of anesthetics."

As you know, Ken got me involved in aerobic exercise by working out *with* me (and in our marriage it was a reverse case of the husband having to overcome the wife's resistance and apathy); we still enjoy doing some of our running together. Additionally, an impressive amount of our mail describes the special pleasures couples find in shared conditioning programs. Let me explain how that works out in terms of coordinating speed and endurance between a man and a woman.

The program Ken recently prescribed for a local Dallas couple is a good example. This husband and wife characterize themselves as having "the pre-50 syndrome": their children are grown and on their own and they feel the need to reduce and get some more youth out of their own lives. Ken had them start together on the 6-week walking/running orientation program. Then they progressed to running a mile and a half in less than 15 minutes to earn 6 points daily—the man with no difficulty, the woman with considerable effort. Now the wife will stay at the 15-minute goal, a good level for her age, but to keep it interesting for her husband, so they can continue running together, he gives her a 30-second headstart; at intervals he works progressively downward in time to giving her a minute, then 90 seconds, then 2 minutes, and so on. Currently, his projected time for the mile-and-a-half is 13 minutes, so he waits with his watch till his wife has been gone for 2 minutes before he starts. This gives both of them an incentive because she tries that much harder to prevent her husband's overtaking her. It's scientific and keeps the program stimulating and challenging for each one.

We know several couples in Dallas for whom exercising together has meant a dramatic and deeply meaningful change in their attitudes toward each other and in their entire outlook on life. My favorite among these is Mary and Ulysses Vlamides, a handsome-looking pair of grandparents in their middle forties. Mary had kept herself in fairly good physical condition, but Uly, a heavy smoker and drinker, was carrying 235 pounds on his 5'10½" frame and working long, stressful hours in his restaurant business. "I thought I was strong enough to change him," Mary says, "but I wasn't. I tried everything—cried, locked him out, nagged. Then it happened that his doctor bought *Aerobics* and told me about it. I read it and passed it on to Uly. Maybe it was those statistics on heart disease, along with fact that our baby granddaughter, the darling of Uly's heart, had recently been born, that put the fear of God into him. But anyway, we started doing stationary running together, and then jogging. We also discovered that the Dallas Cross Country Club, a family-oriented group, had established a running track around a lake in our neighborhood. Uly really took to running and the enthusiasm of the club members affected him, too. He decided he was going to compete in the group's 'Turkey Trot,' an eight-mile race staged at Thanksgiving time. Well, it was pathetic and it was comic and in the end it led to a near miracle."

According to Mary, Uly had never run more than 4 miles at a stretch before he competed in the race, and he turned up for the event wearing tennis shoes, slacks and a sports jacket. He weighed close to 230 pounds. When he got there he was mortified to see lean, keen, experienced runners in their special shoes and track suits. He would have gone home immediately if 20 or so boosters hadn't been around to urge him on. When the results were in, all runners finished the race including Uly—last. As he puts it, "It wasn't too bad until the seventy-year-old man passed me—then I got a lump in my throat."

But the most important consequence of the race was that it created an image for him. The local newspaper and television station covered the event and as the persevering caboose of the group, Uly was interviewed and featured. It was a shot in the arm for him and had a lot to do with his deciding to go on a diet, and to quit smoking and drinking.

In the meantime, Mary, who had begun the aerobics program with her husband simply to encourage him, had fallen off. Now she and their friends watched what was happening to Uly with awe and admiration. Gradually he worked his aerobics program up to running 30 miles a week and worked his weight down to 185 pounds. His vitality, good looks and enthusiasm seemed to increase every day. "I envied his transformation," Mary recalls. "For years I'd nagged him to start taking better care of himself and suddenly there was no stopping him."

In June 1970, about a year after Uly's "rehabilitation" began, he met a coach who told him about the Boston Marathon and that a year of training would prepare him adequately for running in it. Competing in that race in 1971 became his Mecca.

"If I can finish the Boston Marathon," he informed Mary, "I'll take you to Europe."

"Okay," she answered, "we'll make a pact. I'll run the Turkey Trot in November, you do the Boston Marathon in April."

Now both Vlamideses went into serious training, often running late at night after a day's work in their restaurants. Mary would do a mile and a half a day and a weekly LSD run (long slow distance) of 6 miles. Uly worked up to running 50 or 60 miles a week and his weight took a further plunge, into the 170's. Mary lived up to her promise and ran the Turkey Trot, finishing, like her husband, in the caboose position, but equally elated at having completed the race. And then came an unpleasant surprise. Uly learned that his Amateur Athletic Union-certified running experience would not be built up sufficiently to qualify him in time for the Boston Marathon.

No matter. He decided to run in the Dallas Cross Country Club's own marathon in March. And he did. Unexpectedly, so did his wife.

The day of the big event was windy. Uly started his 26-mile endurance test cheered on by his usual group of boosters, Mary among them. The hours passed and the first runners began to cross the finish line. Mary, curious and impatient, suddenly made up her mind to go out with the driver of the pace car to see how Uly was doing. At the 20-mile mark, she found her husband—on the very brink of dropping out.

"It's gone," he gasped, when he saw his wife.

Her instantaneous reply: "Oh, no it's not. You can't quit. I'll get out and run with you."

Wearing a slacks suit and leather sandals instead of running shoes, she climbed out of the car and ran those last 6 windblown miles with Uly. "She talked to me," he remembers. "I used her as a crying towel the whole time and it worked."

"I panicked," Mary says. "And besides, the deal for Europe was still on!"

Uly walked the last mile and his completion time was 4 hours, 18 minutes. The victory belonged to both of them.

The idea of going to Europe that summer became anticlimactic for the Vlamideses, but they plan to attend the Munich Olympics. Uly has since completed "the perfect marathon"—running easily, without straining, the whole distance and completing the race in 3 hours, 45 minutes. They continue to run together—and to look a decade younger than their years.

I'm not suggesting that marathon running is a likely goal for most couples, nor even anything like the amount of time the Vlamideses have come to put into their conditioning program. But what wife wouldn't take the greatest pleasure in knowing she was responsible for her husband's newly found health-through-exercise? What wife wouldn't treasure a gift like the one Uly gave Mary when he told her, "This is the greatest thing you've ever done for me."

YOU'RE AMONG FRIENDS

In an earlier chapter, I mentioned the inspiration that group exercise can provide in helping you to start a conditioning program and stay with it. Banding together to fight a common problem makes a lot of sense—in fact, the T-groups, or therapy groups, that have sprung up all over the country in recent years reflect exactly this tactic. Smokers, calorie counters, students of sensitivity training, and on a graver level, gamblers, drug addicts and alcoholics, have all found strength, motivation, fuel for their willpower and heartening fellowship in working together and supporting each other.

From the very beginning of his aerobics research during his Air Force years, Ken's experience has been that people are highly responsive to group conditioning. The affectionately named Cooper's Poopers' Club ran eagerly and faithfully on their own time, lunch hours and after five p.m. They even designed their own insignia, depicting a bird of the cuckoo family (!) that's native to the Southwest—it's called the roadrunner or chaparral bird and is noted for running with great speed.

If you're overweight, it certainly does make you feel less self-conscious and conspicuous to exercise with others in the same shape rather than on your own. But even more important and morale-lifting, I think, is the simple human contact. My own exercise profile is a potpourri. Sometimes I work out by myself, sometimes with Ken and sometimes, particularly after I've fallen off, the best way for me to reestablish and maintain the everyday routine is to run with other women. Campers and wilderness backpackers know the special rapport, the helping spirit, that surviving in the woods inspires—it's not unlike the camaraderie that comes with sharing and struggling together in a conditioning program.

Another comparison between conditioning and camping is the "tonic" feeling both produce. One night I was with half a dozen women, members of the Dallas Cross Country Club, who exercise together. They got so excited just talking about the way running made them feel that they fairly bubbled. "You sure do get admiration from your husband . . ." "That's right, it's like a short course in how to impress your man . . ." "People need people. One pulls the other. Somehow in a group, extending yourself for that extra twenty or thirty seconds doesn't hurt as much . . ." "You hit age forty, but the idea of aging doesn't bother you. You know you're doing something for yourself . . ." "Right, some women will go and spend a thousand dollars a week at one of those 'beauty farms,' but you don't *think* of needing that when you're running . . ." "If I'm running regularly, I *know* I look good—it shows in my face."

I couldn't write fast enough to capture their effervescence. What I can do, though, is share a letter with you that represents hundreds of similar ones Ken has received from women who are participating in neighborhood exercise groups in every section of the United States. Mrs. Shirley Adcock of Orange, California, speaks for an uncounted but vast sisterhood.

> I do wish you could see what your book has done for us. Three of us had started jogging before it came out, but our program was rather aimless since we didn't know what we should be striving for. We all ended up with painful ankles, since we were running on concrete around the neighborhood. Each of us needed exercise— I personally had just failed my four-hundredth diet and was terribly despondent. One of us weighed more than 170 pounds. One was in her late thirties, one was 40 and I'm 42. Then Aerobics came into being!
>
> Now we run around the local park. The Park Department sent out a man to measure off a mile, mile and

*a half, and 2 miles for us. He put up the markers and
said the department was delighted we were starting
something like that. Now we have the butcher from the
market next to the park, firemen from a nearby station
house, a policeman who used to cruise by early in the
morning and watch us, 3 businessmen, and our "core
group" has increased from 3 women to 8. Everyone is
very earnest—and we have such a feeling of accomplishment when we are done and the day stretches before us,
and we all have energy we didn't think we possessed.*

*I know you're interested in lungs and circulation and
heart and all that stuff, but for us there is the marvelous feeling of a lower dress size, squeals of delight as
the marker on the scale goes down, and the ability to
eat less without dieting. I don't know how to explain
it, but we are all in your debt for Aerobics. My husband now makes the remark, "Oh Lord, here comes the
Messiah with her Bible!" when I bring out your book
to try to entice a new recruit into our bunch, but I note
that he's becoming interested in running, too.*

*If you ever need a picture of a group of sweating,
huffing, puffing females—all with grins on their faces—
please let me know. Also, if this letter can be of help
to you in trying to interest more women in something
they may not consider "genteel" but that can be of
great benefit to them, then by all means use it. As you
said, vigorous exercise may not be a "pretty" pastime—
but what a pretty aftermath we all enjoy!*

15: Typical Questions from Our Mailbox and Audiences

ONE MORNING KEN'S mail brought a question from a correspondent who wanted to know how he could utilize the strength that was presently confined to the area of his belly button. That, needless to say, gave us a belly laugh—and it was *not* a typical query.

In this section I'll give Ken's answers to the questions about aerobics that come up most frequently, some with general relevance and some relating to special situations.

UPHILL DISTANCE

"I live in the mountains of Tennessee and nowhere in my neighborhood is it the least bit flat. In the first week of the walking starter program I should be covering a mile in 15 minutes. Does this apply to uphill distance as well as flat?"

Yes, there's extra benefit to walking up and down hills but the exact amount is hard to quantitate. If the aggregates of uphill and downhill walking are equal, they tend to compensate for each other. However, if the majority of your course is uphill, then the energy requirement is greater. In that case, you can add roughly 2 minutes to each of the time requirements.

MOUNTAIN CLIMBING, WALKING IN HEAVY SNOW

"Is there any way to determine what aerobic points I would earn for several hours of climbing in the mountains? What about hiking in deep snow with heavy boots on?"

Mountain climbing is an excellent way to accumulate points. Once the extra burden of hypoxia (insufficient oxygen) is added to the exercise, the point value rapidly increases. Unfortunately, it's impossible to establish a reliable point system because one can climb so many ways. I can assure you, though, that sustained mountain climbing is worth at least 15 to 20 points an hour. Walking or running in deep snow adds considerable resistance to the exercise and should be worth additional points. Again, this is a difficult activity to quantitate exactly. As a suggestion, double the point value.

UPHILL CYCLING

"My husband and I are cyclists. Our local streets are made up of short blocks, uphill-and-down-dale-style. Thus we're unable to take advantage of downhill runs. Both of us are able to cover the required distance in the given time but it exhausts us. What do you advise?"

This is a true problem that really will reduce your performance. Consequently you can add about 25 percent more time (a 12-minute requirement would be increased to 15 minutes) or you can reduce the distance. I know this is somewhat complicated, but the only alternative is to put your bikes in the car and drive to a reasonably flat stretch of road.

LOW HEART RATE AS HEALTH INDEX

"What evidence is there that a slower heart rate contributes to longer life? Mine is 60 beats a minute and I can hardly get around."

The resting heart rate isn't an absolute indicator of physical fitness. Many people have a very low resting heart rate due to a diseased heart. Only a resting heart rate of 60 that resulted from a regular exercise program could be equated with health.

SPEED VS. DISTANCE

"Two friends and I are actively involved in the aerobics jogging program. We started 2 weeks ago and are already jogging a mile in 11 minutes so we're very enthusiastic over our progress. Our question is, which is more important, achieving the time goal or the distance?"

Ken suggests concentrating more on distance than on speed. Work on achieving your points regardless of the time it takes to earn them. For example, a 2-mile run in less than 16 minutes is worth 10 points whereas a 2-mile walk/run in less than 20 minutes is worth 8 points. The latter performed 3 times a week is worth 24 points and gives you the minimum value. Many women prefer to obtain points only by walking and this is certainly a satisfactory way to develop the training effect.

SIDE ACHE

"I've started the aerobics program and many times I get an ache in my side or stomach when I run. Will this go away when I get into better shape? It doesn't seem serious."

An ache in the side is quite characteristic during the early stages of an exercise program. It's commonly referred to as a stitch and does tend to disappear as you become better conditioned.

HORMONE PILLS

"My question concerns the postmenopausal group who are on estrogen. Does 'the pill' have any effect on an aerobics exercise program?"

You're actually talking about two different kinds of hormone pill. Postmenopausal women who are supplementing their hormone level usually do it with estrogen (which reduces—but doesn't completely resolve—the osteoporosis, or weak-bones, problem that often accompanies aging). The birth-control pill is primarily progesterone rather than estrogen (and has no effect on weak bones). For women who are taking either hormone pill I recommend earning the basic minimum of 24 points a week in their age category.

DIFFICULTY IN STATIONARY RUNNING

"Running in place is the only exercise for me—that is, it's the most practical. Unfortunately, I'm *still* trying to reach and maintain the 2½-minute level. All too soon my legs begin to feel heavy, achy in the muscles and then weak. Afterwards I'm obliged to drop onto my bed for several minutes. Is there a way to overcome this problem?"

In cases where people have considerable difficulty with stationary running, Ken tends to encourage them to switch to an active walking program instead. The trick is to work up to walking between 1.5 and 3 miles a day. When this level is achieved, strength in the legs usually returns.

AEROBIC POINTS FOR DANCING

"I'm convinced that dancing has an aerobic effect. It's fun, of course, but I also believe I gain fitness from it. Many of my women friends enjoy it too; we sweat, and we benefit from it, but we have no way at our disposal to measure the benefit.

"I feel that if the benefits could be measured and charted, we would have a program that (1) we could do at home accompanied by a radio or record player, (2) would be fun, (3) would not be boring because it can be varied and integrated with other aerobic activity, (4) could be engaged in regardless of weather, (5) has aerobic potential plus the bonus of developing grace, poise and rhythm."

Ken is becoming more and more convinced that professional dancers are in exceptionally good physical condition. From contact with classical dancers like ballet master George Balanchine and reading about popular dancers like Juliet Prowse, he knows that they are not only superbly fit in the aerobic sense, but that they depend on vigorous exercise as a means of keeping in the shape necessary to dance professionally. (This is also true of other kinds of performers. Dinah Shore exercises daily. The well-known stage actress Julie Harris told Ken she walks as much as possible and exercises before every appearance to relax and limber up her body.)

Frankly, it just isn't possible to quantitate precisely the oxygen cost of continuous dancing—it can be done in so many ways that measurement really isn't feasible. Purely as an estimate, since Ken has no substantial backup data, he thinks aerobic points might be awarded for a time period of 30 minutes of continuous dancing. See page 154 in the Appendix for a breakdown of points according to the type of dance.

One of the fitness tests might be used to determine the effectiveness of active dancing. After taking at least 10 weeks to build up to earning 24 points a week with dance activity, you could take the test—with appropriate medical clearance if over age 30—to see what fitness category you had achieved.

STATIONARY RUNNING AS PREPARATION FOR DISTANCE RUNNING

"I use the stationary running program and have worked up to an average of 40 points a week. Could you please anwer 2 questions? What is the reason for my inability to run a mile without great difficulty? After all, I can run in place for 20 minutes, about 90 to 100 steps a minute, without any problem. What's the difference? Also, why am I developing flat feet? My tennis shoes supposedly have good support and I wear arch supports."

Stationary running doesn't train the same muscles that long-distance running does. For this reason, people who run in place frequently find it difficult to run a mile or a mile and a half in the required time. However, with a little additional training in distance running, it eventually becomes quite easy for them to meet the minimum requirement for their age. As for foot problems, even with stationary running it's essential to purchase a pair of good cushion-soled track shoes.

HAIRDO SURVIVAL

"When I exercise, I perspire a lot, including my scalp, and the set just vanishes from my hair, leaving it in strings. Why is exercise so hard on hairdos?"

I guess it depends on the individual head of hair, but certainly we hear plenty of complaints from women about deflated coiffures after they've exercised. Some women tell us this reason alone keeps them from getting into a conditioning program. But with inexpensive wigs and hairpieces so easily available in so many becoming styles, the looks of your hair shouldn't be an excuse for not exercising.

Think about how much more your pretty hairstyle will be appreciated if it tops a super-attractive body. Maybe for you the solution will be to wear a short, natural cut that you can shampoo quickly and that doesn't need setting, or to grow your hair long enough to tie back sleekly. For my part, I go to the beauty salon on Friday and enjoy a fancy hairstyle on weekends when I don't exercise. During the rest of the week I try to exercise at a time of day when I'll perspire least. Basically, I don't worry about it. Truly, your hair will be your crowning glory if you have a fit body.

AEROBICS AND SMOKING

Will aerobics help an addictive smoker? Can a smoker enjoy aerobic benefits even if he can't manage to give up his habit? We still get a disappointing number of questions on this subject.

Smoking is known to have a role in heart disease as well as lung disease. Smokers are three times more susceptible to heart attack than nonsmokers. Unfortunately, exercisers who have as few as ten cigarettes a day never reach their maximum performance because the body's ability to carry oxygen from the lungs to the muscles is diminished.

Many people who get into a conditioning program quit it because they find they can't progress beyond a certain point —the smoking limits their lung capacity to that extent!

On the brighter side, exercise becomes a substitute for smoking for other people and they give up tobacco. It's a matter of replacing a destructive habit with a constructive one.

To sum up, people who want to continue smoking should by all means exercise because they badly need to do *something* to offset the effect of tobacco.

AEROBICS AND ALCOHOL

Many men and women enjoy a drink before a meal or at social gatherings and they ask us if taking alcoholic beverages will impair their ability to earn aerobic points and develop a training effect.

As the saying goes, one man's meat is another man's poison. One drink for Mrs. Jones may be the equivalent of three for Miss Smith. So it's impossible for us to make a flat statement, other than that refraining from drinking is the only way we know to ensure no detrimental effect.

When you consider that an ounce and a half of gin, rum, vodka or whiskey costs 150 calories and requires running a mile and one half in 12 minutes or walking 2½ miles in 50 minutes, that may be argument enough in favor of passing up a cocktail.

16: Vigorous, Virtuous, Victorious and (Why Not?) Vainglorious

WHEN KEN LOOKED at my heading for this final chapter, he commented, "What more do you need to say? You've got it all in the title." You'd think he'd remember by now that I almost always have more to say—and in these last few pages it's on motivation.

A strong motivation is certainly the crucial factor in anything people set out to accomplish, and goals and objectives are an enormous help in making us persevere. One of the most exciting things about the aerobics point system is the goal-seeking aspect of it. The progressive levels Ken has established for women are challenging yet entirely feasible, and they're conservatively designed so that if you follow them faithfully you'll keep out of trouble from the standpoint of physical exertion.

The reward for your effort will be *feeling* the "four v's" I strung out above and *knowing* you're using the best method science has devised so far to safeguard your physical health.

Using exercise as preventive therapy isn't a new idea, but rather the revitalization of an old one. Years ago, doctors concentrated on trying to keep people healthy through preventive medicine. But in recent decades, certain diseases have reached epidemic proportions (cardiovascular ones produce more than a million deaths each year) and these diseases attack people at a younger age (heart disease causes death in 1 out of 10 people under 35, 1 out of 3 over 35). Moreover, all sorts of new forms of physical ailments have developed. So doctors have been obliged to devote the larger share of their time to treating the acute process. When the house is on fire you've got to put it out and worry about preventing fires later on.

With the doctor-patient ratio we have in this country—we

need another 50,000 doctors at least—obviously the vast majority of physicians have to spend their time putting out fires. Ken hopes that aerobic therapy will help make doctors *and* the general population think more about preventing fires from happening. If they do, I'm sure in the long run we'll have a better doctor-patient ratio because fewer people will be sick.

The American Health Foundation states that 87,300,000 Americans—almost half the population—suffer from one or more chronic diseases, and it goes on to say, "Ours is the legacy of a medical system that provides too much care too late."

That's very true. That's why the ultimate message of this book is: Don't wait. Please care *now* about your health, while you've still got it. And smile with me over this letter we just received from Mrs. Pat Neumann, the Indiana woman who described her aerobics experience in the first chapter.

> *I'm exercising more slowly these days for guess what reason. Of all things, at the age of 40 and after 15 years of marriage, I'm apparently going to have a baby. We're flabbergasted! I'm not supposed to do anything "strenuous," but thanks to aerobics, running a few miles isn't strenuous for me. When I increase in size I'll switch to swimming.*
>
> *I'm no longer afraid I'll lose my motivation and quit my exercise program. I expect I'll be running all the way until it'll be a padding little jog in my old age. I like the benefits too much.*
>
> *For example, when I told the obstetrician my age, he said, "You mean twenty-nine, don't you?"*
>
> *"No, thirty-nine, I'm thirty-nine," I said, smugly. Ahhhhhhh-robics.*

Appendix: The Point System Expanded

1. WALKING/RUNNING

(at 1/10-Mile Increments)

In measuring a course that starts and finishes in front of their home, many people have found that it is impossible to end on an even mile or half-mile. Consequently, hundreds have asked for a chart that gives the point value for walking and running distances measured in 1/10 miles. The following special chart is in response to this request and gives the point value for walking and running one to five miles at 1/10-mile increments.

1.0 Mile

19:59—14:30 min	1
14:29—12:00 min	2
11:59—10:00 min	3
9:59— 8:00 min	4
7:59— 6:31 min	5
6:30— 5:45 min	6
under 5:45 min	7

1.1 Miles

21:59—15:57 min	1⅛
15:56—13:12 min	2¼
13:11—11:00 min	3⅓
10:59— 8:48 min	4½
8:47— 7:09 min	5½
7:08— 6:20 min	6⅔
under 6:20 min	7¾

1.2 Miles

23:59—17:24 min	1¼
17:23—14:24 min	2½
14:23—12:00 min	3⅔
11:59— 9:36 min	5
9:35— 7:48 min	6
7:47— 6:55 min	7⅓
under 6:55 min	8½

1.3 Miles

25:59—18:51 min	1⅜
18:50—15:36 min	2¾
15:35—13:00 min	4
12:59—10:24 min	5½

1.3 Miles (Cont.)

10:23— 8:27 min	6½
8:26— 7:30 min	8
under 7:30 min	9¼

1.4 Miles

27:59—20:18 min	1½
20:17—16:48 min	2¾
16:47—14:00 min	4½
13:59—11:00 min	6
10:59— 9:06 min	7
9:05— 8:05 min	8⅔
under 8:05 min	10

1.5 Miles

29:59—21:45 min	1½
21:44—18:00 min	3
17:59—15:00 min	4½
14:59—12:00 min	6
11:59— 9:45 min	7½
9:44— 8:40 min	9
under 8:40 min	10½

1.6 Miles

31:59—23:12 min	1⅝
23:11—19:12 min	3¼
19:11—16:00 min	4⅔
15:59—12:48 min	6½
12:47—10:24 min	8
10:23— 9:15 min	9⅔
under 9:15 min	11¼

1. WALKING/RUNNING (CONTINUED)
(at 1/10-Mile Increments)

1.7 Miles

33:59—24:39 min	1¾
24:38—20:24 min	3½
20:23—17:00 min	5
16:59—13:36 min	7
13:35—11:03 min	8½
11:02— 9:50 min	10⅓
under 9:50 min	12

1.8 Miles

35:59—26:06 min	1⅞
26:05—21:36 min	3¾
21:35—18:00 min	5⅓
17:59—14:24 min	7½
14:23—11:42 min	9
11:41—10:25 min	11
under 10:25 min	12¾

1.9 Miles

37:59—27:33 min	1⅞
27:32—22:48 min	3¾
22:47—19:00 min	5⅔
18:59—15:12 min	7½
15:11—12:21 min	9½
12:20—11:00 min	11½
under 11:00 min	13½

2.0 Miles

40:00 min or longer	1
39:59—29:00 min	2
28:59—24:00 min	4
23:59—20:00 min	6
19:59—16:00 min	8
15:59—13:00 min	10
12:59—11:30 min	12
under 11:30 min	14

2.1 Miles

42:00 min or longer	1*
41:59—30:27 min	2⅛
30:26—25:12 min	4¼
25:11—21:00 min	6⅓

2.1 Miles (Cont.)

20:59—16:48 min	8½
16:47—13:39 min	10½
13:38—12:05 min	12⅔
under 12:05 min	14¾

2.2 Miles

44:00 min or longer	1*
43:59—31:54 min	2¼
31:53—26:24 min	4½
26:23—22:00 min	6⅔
21:59—17:36 min	9
17:35—14:18 min	11
14:17—12:40 min	13⅓
under 12:40 min	15½

2.3 Miles

46:00 min or longer	1*
45:59—33:21 min	2⅜
33:20—27:36 min	4¾
27:35—23:00 min	7
22:59—18:24 min	9½
18:23—14:57 min	11½
14:56—13:15 min	14
under 13:15 min	16¼

2.4 Miles

48:00 min or longer	1*
47:59—34:48 min	2½
34:47—28:48 min	4¾
28:47—24:00 min	7⅓
23:59—19:12 min	9½
19:11—15:36 min	12
15:35—13:50 min	14½
under 13:50 min	17

2.5 Miles

50:00 min or longer	1*
49.59—36:15 min	2½
36:14—30:00 min	5
29:59—25:00 min	7½
24:59—20:00 min	10
19:59—16:15 min	12½

* Exercise of sufficient duration to be of cardiovascular benefit. At this speed, ordinarily no training effect would occur. However, the duration is of such extent that a training effect does begin to occur.

1. WALKING/RUNNING (CONTINUED)
(at 1/10-Mile Increments)

2.5 Miles (Cont.)

16:14—14:20 min	15
under 14:20 min	17½

2.6 Miles

52:00 min or longer	1*
51:59—37:42 min	2⅝
37:41—31:12 min	5¼
31:11—26:00 min	7⅔
25:59—20:48 min	10½
20:47—16:54 min	13
16:53—15.00 min	15⅔
under 15:00 min	18¼

2.7 Miles

54:00 min or longer	1*
53:59—39:09 min	2¾
39.08—32:24 min	5½
32:23—27:00 min	8
26:59—21:36 min	11
21:35—17:33 min	13½
17:32—15:35 min	16⅓
under 15:35 min	19

2.8 Miles

56:00 min or longer	1*
55:59—40:36 min	2⅞
40:35—33:36 min	5¾
33:35—28:00 min	8⅓
27:59—22:24 min	11½
22:23—18:12 min	14
18:11—16:10 min	17
under 16:10 min	19¾

2.9 Miles

58:00 min or longer	1*
57:59—42:03 min	2⅞
42:02—34:48 min	5¾
34:47—29:00 min	8⅔
28:59—23:12 min	11½
23:11—18:51 min	14½
18:50—16:45 min	17½
under 16:45 min	20¼

3.0 Miles

1 hr or longer	1½*
59:59—43:30 min	3
43:29—36:00 min	6
35:59—30:00 min	9
29:59—24:00 min	12
23:59—19:30 min	15
19:29—17:15 min	18
under 17:15 min	21

3.1 Miles

1 hr 2:00 min or longer	1½*
1 hr 1:59—44:57 min	3⅛
44:56—37:12 min	6¼
37:11—31:00 min	9⅓
30:59—24:48 min	12½
24:47—20:10 min	15½
20:09—17:50 min	18⅔
under 17:50 min	21¾

3.2 Miles

1 hr 4:00 min or longer	1½*
1 hr 3:59—46:24 min	3¼
46:23—38:24 min	6½
38:23—32:00 min	9⅔
31:59—25:36 min	13
25:35—20:49 min	16
20:48—18:25 min	19⅓
under 18:25 min	22½

3.3 Miles

1 hr 6 min or longer	1½*
1 hr 5:59—47.51 min	3⅜
47:50—39:36 min	6¾
39:35—33:00 min	10
32:59—26:24 min	13½
26:23—21:28 min	16½
21:27—19:00 min	20
under 19:00 min	23¼

3.4 Miles

1 hr 8:00 min or longer	1½*
1 hr 7:59—49:18 min	3⅜

* Exercise of sufficient duration to be of cardiovascular benefit. At this speed, ordinarily no training effect would occur. However, the duration is of such extent that a training effect does begin to occur.

1. WALKING/RUNNING (CONTINUED)

(at 1/10-Mile Increments)

3.4 Miles (Cont.)

49:17—40:48 min	6¾
40:47—34:00 min	10
33:59—27:12 min	13½
27:11—22:07 min	17
22:06—19:35 min	20⅓
under 19:35 min	23¾

3.5 Miles

1 hr 10:00 min or longer	1½*
1 hr 9:59—50:45 min	3½
50:44—42:00 min	7
41:59—35:00 min	10½
34:59—28:00 min	14
27:59—22:45 min	17½
22:44—20:10 min	21
under 20:10 min	24½

3.6 Miles

1 hr 12:00 min or longer	1½*
1 hr 11:59—52:12 min	3⅝
52:11—43:12 min	7¼
43:11—36:00 min	10⅔
35:59—28:48 min	14½
28:47—23:24 min	18
23:23—20:45 min	21⅔
under 20:45 min	25¼

3.7 Miles

1 hr 14:00 min or longer	1½*
1 hr 13:59—53:39 min	3¾
53:38—44:24 min	7½
44:23—37:00 min	11
36:59—29:36 min	15
29:35—24:03 min	18½
24:02—21:15 min	22⅓
under 21:15 min	26

3.8 Miles

1 hr 16:00 min or longer	1½
1 hr 15:59—55:06 min	3⅞
55:05—45:36 min	7¾
45:35—38:00 min	11⅓

3.8 Miles (Cont.)

37:59—30:24 min	15½
30:23—24:42 min	19
24:41—21:50 min	23½
under 21:50 min	26¾

3.9 Miles

1 hr 18:00 min or longer	1½
1 hr 17:59—56:33 min	3⅞
56:32—46:48 min	7¾
46:47—39:00 min	11⅔
38:59—31:12 min	15½
31:11—25:21 min	19½
25:20—22:25 min	23⅔
under 22:25 min	27¼

4.0 Miles

1 hr 20:00 m'1 or longer	2*
1 hr 19:59—58:00 min	4
57:59—48:00 min	8
47:59—40:00 min	12
39:59—32:00 min	16
31:59—26:00 min	20
25:59—23:00 min	24
under 23:00 min	28

4.1 Miles

1 hr 22:00 min or longer	2*
1 hr 21:59—59:27 min	4⅛
59:26—49:12 min	8¼
49:11—41:00 min	12⅓
40:59—32:48 min	16½
32:47—26:39 min	20½
26:38—23:35 min	24⅔
under 23:35 min	28¾

4.2 Miles

1 hr 24:00 min or longer	2*
1 hr 23:59—60:54 min	4¼
60:53—50:24 min	8½
50:23—42:00 min	12⅔
41:59—33.36 min	17
33:35—27:18 min	21

* Exercise of sufficient duration to be of cardiovascular benefit. At this speed, ordinarily no training effect would occur. However, the duration is of such extent that a training effect does begin to occur.

1. WALKING/RUNNING (CONTINUED)
(at 1/10-Mile Increments)

4.2 Miles (Cont.)

27:17—24:10 min	25⅓
under 24:10 min	29½

4.3 Miles

1 hr 26:00 min or longer	2*
1 hr 25:59—1 hr 2:21 min	4⅜
1 hr 2:20—51:36 min	8¾
51:35—43:00 min	13
42:59—34:24 min	17½
34:23—27:57 min	21½
27:56—24:45 min	26
under 24:45 min	30¼

4.4 Miles

1 hr 28:00 min or longer	2*
1 hr 27:59—1 hr 3:48 min	4½
1 hr 3:47—52:48 min	8¾
52:47—44:00 min	13⅓
43:59—35:12 min	17½
35:11—28:36 min	22
28:35—25:20 min	26⅓
under 25:20 min	31

4.5 Miles

1 hr 30:00 min or longer	2*
1 hr 29:59—1 hr 5:15 min	4½
1 hr 5:14—54:00 min	9
53:59—45:00 min	13½
44:59—36:00 min	18
35:59—29:15 min	22½
29:14—25:55 min	27
under 25:55 min	31½

4.6 Miles

1 hr 32:00 min or longer	2*
1 hr 31:59—1 hr 6:42 min	4⅝
1 hr 6:41—55:12 min	9¼
55:11—46:00 min	13⅔
45:59—36:48 min	18½
36:47—29:54 min	23
29:53—26:30 min	27⅔
under 26:30 min	32¼

4.7 Miles

1 hr 34:00 min or longer	2*
1 hr 33:59—1 hr 8:09 min	4¾
1 hr 8:08—56:24 min	9½
56:23—47:00 min	14
46:59—37:36 min	19
37:35—30:33 min	23½
30:32—27:00 min	28⅓
under 27:00 min	33

4.8 Miles

1 hr 36:00 min or longer	2*
1 hr 35:59—1 hr 9:36 min	4⅞
1 hr 9:35—57:36 min	9¾
57:35—48:00 min	14⅓
47:59—38:24 min	19½
38:23—31:12 min	24
31:11—27:35 min	29
under 27:35 min	33¾

4.9 Miles

1 hr 38:00 min or longer	2*
1 hr 37:59—1 hr 11:03 min	4⅞
1 hr 11:02—58:48 min	9¾
58:47—49:00 min	14⅔
48:59—39:12 min	19½
39:11—31:51 min	24½
31:50—28:10 min	29½
under 28:10 min	34¼

5.0 Miles

1 hr 40:00 min or longer	2½*
1 hr 39:59—1 hr 12:30 min	5
1 hr 12:29—1 hr	10
59:59—50:00 min	15
49:59—40:00 min	20
39:59—32:30 min	25
32:29—28:45 min	30
under 28:45 min	35

* Exercise of sufficient duration to be of cardiovascular benefit. At this speed, ordinarily no training effect would occur. However, the duration is of such extent that a training effect does begin to occur.

1. WALKING/RUNNING (CONTINUED)

(at 1/2-Mile Increments)

5.5 Miles

1 hr 50:00 min or longer	2½*
1 hr 49:59—1 hr 19:45 min	5½
1 hr 19:44—1 hr 6:00 min	11
1 hr 5:59—55:00 min	16½
54:59—44:00 min	22
43:59—35:45 min	27½
35:44—31:35 min	33
under 31:35 min	38½

6.0 Miles

2 hrs or longer	3*
1 hr 59:59—1 hr 27:00 min	6
1 hr 26:59—1 hr 12:00 min	12
1 hr 11:59—1 hr	18
59:59—48:00 min	24
47:59—39:00 min	30
38:59—34:30 min	36
under 34:30 min	42

6.5 Miles

2 hrs 10:00 min or longer	3*
2 hrs 9:59—1 hr 34:15 min	6½
1 hr 34:14—1 hr 18:00 min	13
1 hr 17:59—1 hr 5:00 min	19½
1 hr 4:59—52:00 min	26
51:59—42:15 min	32½
42:14—37:22 min	39
under 37:22 min	45½

7.0 Miles

2 hrs 20:00 min or longer	3½*
2 hrs 19:59—1 hr 41:30 min	7
1 hr 41:29—1 hr 24:00 min	14
1 hr 23:59—1 hr 10:00 min	21
1 hr 9:59—56:00 min	28
55:59—45:30 min	35
45:29—40:15 min	42
under 40:15 min	49

7.5 Miles

2 hrs 30:00 min or longer	3½*
2 hrs 29:59—1 hr 48:45 min	7½
1 hr 48:44—1 hr 30:00 min	15
1 hr 29:59—1 hr 15:00 min	22½
1 hr 14:59—1 hr	30
59:59—48:45 min	37½
48:44—43:10 min	45
under 43:10 min	52½

8.0 Miles

2 hrs 40:00 min or longer	4
2 hrs 39:59—1 hr 56:00 min	8
1 hr 55:59—1 hr 36:00 min	16
1 hr 35:59—1 hr 20:00 min	24
1 hr 19:59—1 hr 4:00 min	32
1 hr 3:59—52:00 min	40
51:59—46:00 min	48
under 46:00 min	56

8.5 Miles

2 hrs 50:00 min or longer	4*
2 hrs 49:59—2 hrs 3:15 min	8½
2 hrs 3:14—1 hr 42:00 min	17
1 hr 41:59—1 hr 25:00 min	25½
1 hr 24:59—1 hr 8:00 min	34
1 hr 7:59—55:15 min	42½
55:14—48:50 min	51
under 48:50 min	59½

9.0 Miles

3 hrs or longer	4½*
2 hrs 59:59—2 hrs 10:30 min	9
2 hrs 10:29—1 hr 48:00 min	18
1 hr 47:59—1 hr 30:00 min	27
1 hr 29:59—1 hr 12:00 min	36
1 hr 11:59—58:30 min	45
58:29—51:45 min	54
under 51:45 min	63

* Exercise of sufficient duration to be of cardiovascular benefit. At this speed, ordinarily no training effect would occur. However, the duration is of such extent that a training effect does begin to occur.

1. WALKING/RUNNING (CONTINUED)
(at 1/2-Mile Increments)

9.5 Miles

3 hrs 10:00 min or longer	4½*
3 hrs 9:59—2 hrs 17:45 min	9½
2 hrs 17:44—1 hr 54:00 min	19
1 hr 53:59—1 hr 35:00 min	28½
1 hr 34:59—1 hr 16:00 min	38
1 hr 15:59—1 hr 1:45 min	47½
1 hr 1:44—54:40 min	57
under 54:40 min	66½

10.0 Miles

3 hrs 20:00 min or longer	5*
3 hrs 19:59—2 hrs 25:00 min	10
2 hrs 24:59—2 hrs	20
1 hr 59:59—1 hr 40:00 min	30
1 hr 39:59—1 hr 20:00 min	40
1 hr 19:59—1 hr 5:00 min	50
1 hr 4:59—57:30 min	60
under 57:30 min	70

12.5 Miles

3 hrs 1:15—2 hrs 30:00 min	25
2 hrs 29:59—2 hrs 5:00 min	37½
2 hrs 4:59—1 hr 40:00 min	50
1 hr 39:59—1 hr 21:15 min	62½
under 1 hr 21:15 min	75

15 Miles

3 hrs 37:28 min—3 hrs	30
2 hrs 59:59—2 hrs 30:00 min	45
2 hrs 29:59—2 hrs	60
1 hr 59:59—1 hr 37:30 min	75
under 1 hr 37:30 min	90

20.0 Miles

4 hrs 49:59 min—4 hrs	40
3 hrs 59:59—3 hrs 20:00 min	60
3 hrs 19:59—2 hrs 40:00 min	80
2 hrs 39:59—2 hrs 10:00 min	100
under 2 hrs 10:00 min	120

25.0 Miles

6 hrs 2:25 min—5 hrs	50
4 hrs 59:59—4 hrs 10:00 min	75
4 hrs 9:59—3 hrs 20:00 min	100
3 hrs 19:59—2 hrs 42:30 min	125
under 2 hrs 42:30 min	150

* Exercise of sufficient duration to be of cardiovascular benefit. At this speed, ordinarily no training effect would occur. However, the duration is of such extent that a training effect does begin to occur.

2. ROPE SKIPPING

DURATION (minutes)	POINTS	DURATION (minutes)	POINTS	DURATION (minutes)	POINTS
2:30	¾	9:00	2⅔	15:00	4½
3:00	1	10:00	3	16:00	5¼
4:00	1¼	11:00	3⅓	17:00	6
5:00	1½	12:00	3⅔	17:30	6½
6:00	1⅔	12:30	3¾	18:00	6¾
7:00	2	13:00	4	19:00	7½
7:30	2¼	14:00	4⅓	20:00	8
8:00	2⅓				

Skip with both feet together or step over the rope alternating feet, skipping at a frequency of 70–80 steps per minute.

3. STAIR CLIMBING

(10 steps; 6-7" in height; 25°-30° incline)

ROUND TRIPS—AVERAGE NUMBER PER MINUTE

TIME (minutes)	5	6	7	8	9	10
3:00	—	—	—	—	—	2½
3:30	—	—	—	—	2	—
4:00	—	—	1½	1¾	—	3¼
4:30	—	—	—	—	2¾	—
5:00	½	1	1¾	—	—	4
5:30	—	1¼	—	2½	3½	—
6:00	¾	—	2	—	—	4¾
6:30	—	1½	—	3	4¼	—
7:00	1	—	2¼	—	—	5½
7:30	—	1¾	—	3½	4½	—
8:00	1¼	—	2¾	—	—	6½
8:30	—	2	—	3¾	5½	—
9:00	1½	—	3	4	5¾	7¼
9:30	—	2¼	—	4¼	6	—
10:00	1¾	—	3¼	4½	6½	8
10:30	—	—	3½	4¾	6¾	—
11:00	2	2½	3¾	5	7	8¾
11:30	—	—	—	5¼	7¼	—
12:00	2¼	2¾	4	5½	7½	9½
12:30	—	—	—	5¾	7¾	—
13:00	2½	3	4¼	6	8	10¼
13:30	—	—	—	6¼	8¼	—
14:00	2¾	3¼	4½	6½	8½	11
14:30	—	—	—	6¾	8¾	—
15:00	3	3½	4¾	—	—	—

4. SWIMMING

200 Yards		550 Yards	
6:40 min or longer	0	18:20 min or longer	1*
6.39— 5:00 min	1	18:19—13:45 min	3½
4:59— 3:20 min	1½	13:44— 9:10 min	4½
under 3:20 min	2½	under 9:10 min	7

250 Yards		600 Yards	
8:20 min or longer	0	20:00 min or longer	1½*
8:19— 6:15 min	1¼	19:59—15:00 min	4
6:14— 4:10 min	2	14:59—10:00 min	5
under 4:10 min	3	under 10:00 min	7½

300 Yards		650 Yards	
10:00 min or longer	1*	21:40 min or longer	1½*
9:59— 7:30 min	1½	21:39—16:15 min	4
7:29— 5:00 min	2½	16:14—10:50 min	5½
under 5:00 min	3½	under 10:50 min	8

350 Yards		700 Yards	
11:40 min or longer	1*	23:20 min or longer	1½*
11:39— 8:45 min	2	23:19—17:30 min	4½
8:44— 5:50 min	3	17:29—11:40 min	6
under 5:50 min	4½	under 11:40 min	8½

400 Yards		750 Yards	
13:20 min or longer	1*	25:00 min or longer	1½*
13:19—10:00 min	2½	24:59—18:45 min	4¾
9:59— 6:40 min	3½	18:44—12:30 min	6½
under 6:40 min	5	under 12:30 min	9½

450 Yards		800 Yards	
15:00 min or longer	1*	26:40 min or longer	1½*
14:59—11:15 min	3	26:39—20:00 min	5
11:14— 7:30 min	4	19:59—13:20 min	6½
under 7:30 min	5½	under 13:20 min	10

500 Yards		850 Yards	
16:40 min or longer	1*	28:20 min or longer	1½*
16:39—12:30 min	3	28:19—21:15 min	5¼
12:29— 8:20 min	4	21:14—14:10 min	7
under 8:20 min	6	under 14:10 min	10½

* Exercise of sufficient duration to be of cardiovascular benefits. At this speed, ordinarily no traning effect would occur. However, the duration is of such extent that a training effect does begin to occur.

4. SWIMMING (CONTINUED)

900 Yards

30:00 min or longer	2*
29:59—22:30 min	5½
22:29—15:00 min	7½
under 15:00 min	11¼

950 Yards

31:40 min or longer	2*
31:39—23:15 min	5¾
23:14—15:50 min	8
under 15:50 min	12

1000 Yards

33:20 min or longer	2*
33:19—25:00 min	6¼
24:59—16:40 min	8½
under 16:40 min	12½

1100 Yards

36:40 min or longer	2*
36:39—27:30 min	7
27:29—18:20 min	9
under 18:20 min	13¾

1200 Yards

40:00 min or longer	2½*
39:59—30:00 min	7½
29:59—20:00 min	10
under 20:00 min	15

1300 Yards

43:20 min or longer	2½*
43:19—32:30 min	8
32:29—21:40 min	11
under 21:40 min	16¼

1400 Yards

46:40 min or longer	2½*
46:39—35:00 min	8¾

1400 Yards (Cont.)

34:59—23:20 min	11½
under 23:20 min	17½

1500 Yards

50:00 min or longer	3*
49:59—37:30 min	9½
37:29—25:00 min	12½
under 25:00 min	18¾

1600 Yards

53:20 min or longer	3*
53:19—40:00 min	10
39:59—26:40 min	13¼
under 26:40 min	20

1700 Yards

56:40 min or longer	3*
56:39—42:30 min	10½
42:29—28:20 min	14
under 28:20 min	21¼

1800 Yards

1 hr or longer	3½*
59:59—45:00 min	11
44:59—30:00 min	15
under 30:00 min	22½

1900 Yards

1 hr 3:20 min or longer	3½*
1 hr 3:19—47:30 min	12
47:29—31:40 min	15¾
under 31:40 min	23¾

2000 Yards

1 hr 6:40 min or longer	3½*
1 hr 6:39—50:00 min	12½
49:59—33:20 min	16½
under 33:20 min	25

ADDITIONAL COMMENTS:
Points calculated on overhand crawl, i.e., 9.0 Kcal per min. Breaststroke is less demanding: 7.0 Kcal per min. Backstroke, a little more: 8.0 Kcal per min. Butterfly, most demanding: 12.0 Kcal per min.

* Exercise of sufficient duration to be of cardiovascular benefit. At this speed, ordinarily no training effect would occur. However, the duration is of such extent that a training effect does begin to occur.

5. CYCLING

INSTRUCTIONS:
1. Points determined considering equal uphill and downhill course.
2. Points determined considering equal time with and against the wind.
3. For cycling a one-way course constantly against a wind exceeding 5 mph, add ½ point per mile to the total point value.

2.0 Miles

12 min or longer	0
11:59— 8:00 min	1
7:59— 6:00 min	2
under 6:00 min	3

3.0 Miles

18 min or longer	0
17:59—12:00 min	1½
11:59— 9:00 min	3
under 9:00 min	4½

4.0 Miles

21 min or longer	0
23:59—16:00 min	2
15:59—12:00 min	4
under 12:00 min	6

5.0 Miles

30 min or longer	1*
29:59—20:00 min	2½
19:59—15:00 min	5
under 15:00 min	7½

6.0 Miles

36 min or longer	1*
35:59—24:00 min	3
23:59—18:00 min	6
under 18:00 min	9

7.0 Miles

42 min or longer	1½*
41:59—28:00 min	3½
27:59—21:00 min	7
under 21:00 min	10½

8.0 Miles

48 min or longer	1½*
47:59—32:00 min	4

8.0 Miles (Cont.)

31:59—24:00 min	8
under 24:00 min	12

9.0 Miles

54 min or longer	2*
53:59—36:00 min	4½
35:59—27:00 min	9
under 27:00 min	13½

10.0 Miles

1 hr or longer	2*
59:59—40:00 min	5
39:59—30:00 min	10
under 30:00 min	15

11.0 Miles

1 hr 6 min or longer	2½*
1 hr 5:59 min—44:00 min	5½
43:59—33:00 min	11
under 33:00 min	16½

12.0 Miles

1 hr 12 min or longer	2½*
1 hr 11:59 min—48:00 min	6
47:59—36:00 min	12
under 36:00 min	18

13.0 Miles

1 hr 18 min or longer	3*
1 hr 17:59 min—52:00 min	6½
51:59—39:00 min	13
under 39:00 min	19½

14.0 Miles

1 hr 24 min or longer	3*
1 hr 23:59 min—56:00 min	7
55:59—42:00 min	14
under 42:00 min	21

* Exercise of sufficient duration to be of cardiovascular benefit. At this speed, ordinarily no training effect would occur. However, the duration is of such extent that a training effect does begin to occur.

5. CYCLING (CONTINUED)

15.0 Miles

1 hr 30 min or longer	3½*
1 hr 29:59 min—1 hr	7½
59:59—45:00 min	15
under 45:00 min	22½

19.0 Miles

1 hr 54 min or longer	4½*
1 hr 53:59 min—1 hr 16 min	9½
1 hr 15:59 min—57:00 min	19
under 57:00 min	28½

16.0 Miles

1 hr 36 min or longer	3½*
1 hr 35:59 min—1 hr 4 min	8
1 hr 3:59 min—48:00 min	16
under 48:00 min	24

20.0 Miles

2 hrs or longer	4½*
1 hr 59:59 min—1 hr 20 min	10
1 hr 19:59 min—1 hr	20
under 1 hr	30

17.0 Miles

1 hr 42 min or longer	4*
1 hr 41:59 min—1 hr 8 min	8½
1 hr 7:59 min—51:00 min	17
under 51:00 min	25½

25.0 Miles

2 hrs 30 min or longer	6*
2 hrs 29:59 min—1 hr 40 min	12½
1 hr 39:59 min—1 hr 15 min	25
under 1 hr 15:00 min	37½

18.0 Miles

1 hr 48 min or longer	4*
1 hr 47:59 min—1 hr 12 min	9
1 hr 11:59 min—54:00 min	18
under 54:00 min	27

30.0 Miles

3 hrs or longer	7*
2 hrs 59:59 min—2 hrs	15
1 hr 59:59 min—1 hr 30 min	30
under 1 hr 30:00 min	45

* Exercise of sufficient duration to be of cardiovascular benefit. At this speed, ordinarily no training effect would occur. However, the duration is of such extent that a training effect does begin to occur.

6. STATIONARY CYCLING

(assuming enough resistance to raise the pulse to at least 140, measured immediately after exercise)

Time (minutes)	Average Speed (m.p.h.) 10	12	15	17½	20	25
2:30	—	—	—	—	—	—
3:00	—	—	—	—	—	—
4:00	—	—	½	—	1	—
5:00	—	½	—	—	1¼	2
6:00	½	—	¾	—	1½	2⅛
7:00	—	—	—	1	1¾	2¼
7:30	—	¾	—	1⅛	1⅞	2⅜
8:00	—	—	1	1¼	2	2½
9:00	¾	—	—	1⅜	2¼	2¾
10:00	—	1	1¼	1⅜	2½	3
11:00	—	—	—	1½	2⅝	3¼
12:00	1	—	1⅜	1⅝	2¾	3½
12:30	—	1¼	1½	1⅞	—	3⅝
13:00	—	—	—	1⅞	2⅞	3¾
14:00	—	—	1¾	2	3	4
15:00	1¼	1½	—	2⅛	3⅛	4¼
16:00	—	—	2	2¼	3¼	4½
17:00	—	—	—	2⅜	3⅜	4¾
17:30	—	1¾	—	2½	3½	4⅞
18:00	1½	—	2¼	2⅝	3⅝	5
19:00	—	—	—	2¾	3¾	5⅓
20:00	—	2	2½	2⅞	3⅞	5⅔
21:00	1¾	—	—	3	4	6
22:00	—	—	2¾	3¼	4⅛	6½
22:30	—	2¼	—	—	4½	6⅝
23:00	—	—	—	3⅜	4⅜	6¾
24:00	2	—	3	3½	4½	7
25:00	—	2½	—	3¾	4⅝	7½
26:00	—	—	3¼	4	4⅞	7¾
27:00	2¼	—	—	4¼	5	8
28:00	—	2¾	3½	4½	5⅛	8½
29:00	—	—	—	4¾	5⅜	8¾
30:00	2½	3	3¾	5	5½	9

7. POINT VALUE FOR STATIONARY RUNNING

TIME (minutes)	*60-70 STEPS/MIN	POINTS	*70-80 STEPS/MIN	POINTS	*80-90 STEPS/MIN	POINTS	*90-100 STEPS/MIN	POINTS	*100-110 STEPS/MIN	POINTS
2:30			175-200	¾	200-225	1	225-250	1¼	250-275	1½
5:00	300-350	1¼	350-400	1½	400-450	2	450-500	2½	500-550	3
7:30			525-600	2¼	600-675	3	675-750	3¾	750-825	4½
10:00	600-700	2½	700-800	3	800-900	4	900-1000	5	1000-1100	6
12:30			875-1000	3¾	1000-1125	5	1125-1250	6¼	1250-1375	7½
15:00	900-1050	3¾	1050-1200	4½	1200-1350	6	1350-1500	7½	1500-1650	9
17:30			1225-1400	5¼	1400-1575	7	1575-1750	8¾	1750-1925	10½
20:00	1200-1400	5	1400-1600	6	1600-1800	8	1800-2000	10	2000-2200	12
22:30			1575-1800	6¾	1800-2025	9	2025-2250	11¼	2250-2475	13½
25:00	1500-1750	6¼	1750-2000	7½	2000-2250	10	2250-2500	12½	2500-2750	15
27:30			1925-2200	8¼	2200-2475	11	2475-2750	13¾	2750-3025	16½
30:00	1800-2100	7½	2100-2400	9	2400-2700	12	2700-3000	15	3000-3300	18

* Count only when the left foot hits the floor. Knees must be brought up in front raising the feet at least eight inches from the floor.

8. ADDITIONAL EXERCISES

EXERCISE	DURATION	POINTS	COMMENTS
Badminton	1 game	1½	Singles; players of equal
	2 games	3	ability; length of game,
	3 games	4½	20 minutes
Dancing *			
Square	30 min	2½	Count only the time you
Polka	30 min	2½	are actively dancing
Waltz	30 min	1½	
Modern	30 min	1½	
Watusi,			
Jerk, etc.	30 min	2	
Fencing	10 min	1	
	20 min	2	
	30 min	3	
Golf	9 holes	1½	No motorized carts
	18 holes	3	
Lacrosse and	20 min	3	Count only the time in
Soccer	40 min	6	which you are actively
	60 min	9	participating
Rowing	6 min	1	2 oars, 20 strokes a min-
	18 min	3	ute
	36 min	6	
Skating	15 min	1	Either ice or roller skat-
	30 min	2	ing. For speed skating
	60 min	3	triple the point value
Skiing	30 min	3	Water or snow skiing
	60 min	6	For cross-country snow
	90 min	9	skiing triple the point
			value
Tennis	1 set	1½	Singles; players of equal
	2 sets	3	ability; length of set 20
	3 sets	4½	minutes
Volleyball	15 min	1	
	30 min	2	
	60 min	4	
Walking	½ mile (10:00)	1	
Pushing a stroller	1 mile (20:00)	2	Containing a 15- to 30-
or baby carriage	1½ miles (30:00)	3	pound child

* Point values estimated.

EXERCISE COMBINATIONS TOTALING 24 POINTS

EXERCISE	DISTANCE	DURATION	WEEKDAYS	POINTS	
Rope Skipping	———	13:00	M, Thu	8	
Stair Climbing	———	12:00	Tues, Fri	8	A
Walking	2.0 miles	29:00	Sat, Sun	8	
Walking	1.0 miles	14:00	2X/day, M, W, F	12	
Stationary cycling	———	21:00	Sun	6	B
Swimming	700 yds.	17:00	Sat	6	
Walking	2.0 miles	29:00	Mon-Fri	8	
Tennis	———	3 sets	Wed-Sun	9	C
Cycling	7.0 miles	27:00	Sat	7	
Jogging	1.5 miles	14:45	Mon-Fri	12	
Tennis	———	3 sets	Wed, Sun	9	D
Golf	———	18 holes	Sat	3	
Walking	2.5 miles	29:00	Mon, Wed	15	
Skiing	———	60:00	Sun	6	E
Dancing (Jerk)	———	60:00	Fri, Sat	4	

A. For the housewife with a park nearby.
B. For the woman who wants a well-rounded program and can afford a stationary bicycle.
C. For the tennis player who owns a bicycle.
D. For the avid exercise enthusiast.
E. For the dating girl.

HIGH ALTITUDE COMPENSATION CHART

POINT VALUE FOR WALKING AND RUNNING
ONE MILE AT VARIOUS ALTITUDES

1.0 Mile	Standard	5,000 Feet	Points
	19:59–14:30 min	20:29–15:00 min	1
	14:29–12:00 min	14:59–12:30 min	2
	11:59–10:00 min	12:29–10:30 min	3
	9:59– 8:00 min	10:29– 8:30 min	4
	7:59– 6:30 min	8:29– 7:00 min	5
	Under 6:30 min	Under 7:00 min	6
	8,000 Feet	12,000 Feet	Points
	20:59–15:30 min	21:29–16:30 min	1
	15:29–13:00 min	16:29–14:00 min	2
	12:59–11:00 min	13:59–12:00 min	3
	10:59– 9:00 min	11:59–10:00 min	4
	8:59– 7:30 min	9:59– 8:30 min	5
	Under 7:30 min	Under 8:30 min	6

CALORIE AND EXERCISE EQUIVALENTS FOR POPULAR FOODS AND BEVERAGES
(see page 160 for roman numeral exercise equivalent)

FOOD	SIZE/SERVING	APPROXI-MATE CALORIES	EXERCISE
Almonds	9-10 whole	70	II
Apple	2½" diameter	70	II
Apple, baked with sugar	1 large	200	V
Applesauce, sweetened	½ cup	115	III
Apricots			
canned in water	½ cup	45	I
canned in syrup	½ cup	110	III
Apricots, dried	½ cup, 20 small halves	120	III
Asparagus	6 spears	20	I
Avocado	½ average	185	IV
Bacon, fried	2 slices	90	II
Banana	1 average, 6" x 1½"	80	II
Beans, baked with pork in tomato sauce	½ cup	160	IV
Beans (green, wax, or yellow)	½ cup	15	I
Beans, lima	½ cup	130	III
Beef			
corned, canned	3 ounces	185	IV
hamburger, reg.	3 ounces	245	V
oven roast	3 ounces, lean	200	V
pot roast	3 ounces, lean	165	IV
steak	3 ounces, lean	175	IV
Blueberries	½ cup, fresh	45	I
Bologna	2 ounces, all meat	170	IV
Bread			
white	1 slice, 16 slices per loaf	75	II
whole-wheat	1 slice, 16 slices per loaf	70	II
rye	1 slice, 16 slices per loaf	70	II
Broccoli	½ cup	30	I
Butter	1 pat, 16 per ¼ pound	50	II
Cake			
chocolate with chocolate icing	2" wedge of 10" layer cake	345	VII
plain cake without icing	3" x 2" x 1½" slice	155	IV
pound cake	2¾" x 3" x ⅝" slice	140	III
Candies			
caramels	3 medium	115	III
chocolate creams	2 or 3 small	110	III
fudge, milk chocolate	1 ounce	120	III
hard candy	1 ounce	110	III
milk chocolate	1-ounce bar	150	IV
Cantaloupe	½ melon, 5" diameter	60	II
Carrot	5½" x 1" carrot	20	I

CALORIE AND EXERCISE EQUIVALENTS FOR POPULAR FOODS AND BEVERAGES (CONTINUED)

FOOD	SIZE/SERVING	APPROXIMATE CALORIES	EXERCISE
Celery	Two 8" stalks	10	I
Cereal			
Corn Flakes	1 cup	95	II
Oatmeal	1 cup	130	III
Wheat flakes	1 cup	105	III
Cheese			
American, processed	1 ounce	105	III
Cheddar, natural	1 ounce	115	III
cottage, creamed	1 ounce	30	I
Swiss	1 ounce	105	III
Cherries			
sweet, fresh	½ cup	40	I
sweet, canned with syrup	½ cup	105	III
Chicken	¼ small, broiled	185	IV
Cookies	1 average	30	I
Corn	½ cup	70	II
Crab	½ cup, canned	85	II
Crackers			
graham	4 squares	55	II
rye wafers	2	45	I
saltines	Two, 2" square	35	I
Cucumber	¾" slice	5	I
Custard, baked	½ cup	140	III
Egg	1 large	80	II
Frankfurter	1 average	155	IV
	1 with roll	245	V
Fruit cocktail	½ cup with syrup	100	III
Gelatin dessert	½ cup	70	II
Grapefruit	Half of 4¼" fruit	55	II
	½ cup, canned with water	35	I
	½ cup, canned with syrup	90	II
Gum, chewing	1 stick	10	I
Ham	3 ounces lean	160	IV
Honeydew melon	½ fresh	50	II
Ice cream	½ cup	145	III
	soda, large	455	X
Ice milk	½ cup	110	III
Jams, Jellies	1 tablespoon	55	II
Lamb	3 ounces, lean	160	IV
Lemonade	8-ounce glass	110	III
Lettuce	2 large leaves	10	I
Liver, beef	3 ounces	195	IV
Macaroni	¾ cup, plain	115	III
	¾ cup, with cheese	360	VIII

CALORIE AND EXERCISE EQUIVALENTS FOR POPULAR FOODS AND BEVERAGES
(CONTINUED)

FOOD	SIZE/SERVING	APPROXIMATE CALORIES	EXERCISE
Margarine	1 pat, 16 per ¼ pound	50	II
Milk			
whole	1 cup	160	IV
buttermilk	1 cup	90	II
half-and-half	1 tablespoon	20	I
skim	1 cup	90	II
chocolate	1 cup	210	V
chocolate milkshake	12 ounces	500	X
Muffin			
corn	2¾" diameter	150	IV
English	3½" diameter	135	III
Noodles	¾ cup	150	IV
Oil, salad	1 tablespoon	125	III
Orange juice	½ cup	55	II
Orange	3" fruit	75	II
Pancake	4" cake	55	II
Peach	2" fruit, fresh	35	I
	½ cup, canned in syrup	100	III
Peanuts	2 tablespoons	105	III
Peanut butter	1 tablespoon	95	II
Pear	3" x 2½" fruit	100	III
Peas	½ cup	60	II
Pickle			
dill	1¾" x 4"	15	I
sweet	¾" x 1¾"	30	I
Pie			
fruit	⅛ of 9" pie	300	VII
lemon meringue	⅛ of 9" pie	270	VI
pecan	⅛ of 9" pie	430	IX
Pineapple	½ cup, fresh	40	I
	½ cup, canned	100	III
Plum	2" fruit, fresh	25	I
	½ cup, canned	100	III
Popcorn	1 cup	40	I
Pork	3 ounces, lean	230	V
Potato chips	10 medium	115	III
Potato			
baked	2½", 5 ounces	90	II
French-fried	Ten 2"-long pieces	155	IV
mashed	½ cup	90	II
sweet	5" x 2", 6 ounces	155	IV
Pretzels	5 small sticks	20	I
Prunes	½ cup, unsweetened	150	IV
Radishes	4 small	5	I

CALORIE AND EXERCISE EQUIVALENTS FOR POPULAR FOODS AND BEVERAGES (CONTINUED)

FOOD	SIZE/SERVING	APPROXI- MATE CALORIES	EXERCISE
Raisins	½ cup	230	V
Rice, cooked	¾ cup	140	III
Salad dressing			
blue-cheese	1 tablespoon	75	II
French	1 tablespoon	65	II
low-calorie	1 tablespoon	15	I
mayonnaise	1 tablespoon	100	III
Thousand Island	1 tablespoon	125	III
Salmon	3 ounces, canned	120	III
Sausage, pork	2 ounces	270	VI
Sherbet	½ cup	130	III
Shrimps	3 ounces, 17 medium, canned	100	III
Soft drink			
cola-type	12-ounce can	145	III
fruit flavors	12-ounce can	170	IV
ginger ale	12-ounce can	115	III
root beer	12-ounce can	150	IV
Soup			
bouillon	1 cup	30	I
chicken noodle	1 cup	60	II
cream of mushroom	1 cup	135	III
minestrone	1 cup	105	III
tomato	1 cup, made with water	90	II
tomato	1 cup, made with milk	170	IV
Spaghetti			
plain	¾ cup	115	III
with tomato sauce	¾ cup	195	IV
with meatballs	¾ cup	250	VI
Spinach	½ cup	20	I
Strawberries	½ cup, fresh	30	I
	½ cup, frozen	140	III
Sugar	1 teaspoon	15	I
Tomato juice	½ cup	20	I
Tomatoes	½ cup	25	I
Tuna	3 ounces, canned	170	IV
Turkey	3 ounces, light meat	150	IV
	3 ounces, dark meat	175	IV
Veal	3 ounces, lean	185	IV
Waffle	1 average	210	V
Watermelon	one 2-pound wedge	115	III
Yogurt	1 cup, plain	120	III
	1 cup, with fruit	260	VI

EXERCISE SELECTOR FOR BURNING UP SPECIFIC CALORIC AMOUNTS

I
Exercises Burning up to 50 Calories

Walk ½ mile in 7:30 min
Walk/jog ¼ mile in 3:00 min
Swim 250 yards in 7:30 min
Cycle 1½ miles in 9:00 min

II
Exercises Burning 50–99 Calories

Walk 1 mile in 15:00 min
Walk/jog ¾ mile in 9:00 min
Run ¾ mile in 6:00 min
Swim 450 yards in 15:00 min
Cycle 3 miles in 18:00 min

III
Exercises Burning 100–149 Calories

Walk 1½ miles in 30:00 min
Walk/jog 1 mile in 12:00 min
Run 1 mile in 8:00 min
Swim 900 yards in 30:00 min
Cycle 3 miles in 12:00 min

IV
Exercises Burning 150–199 Calories

Walk 2½ miles in 50:00 min
Walk/jog 1½ miles in 18:00 min
Run 1½ miles in 12:00 min
Swim 1,500 yards in 50:00 min
Cycle 4½ miles in 18:00 min

V
Exercises Burning 200–249 Calories

Walk 3 miles in 45:00 min
Walk/jog 2 miles in 24:00 min
Run 2 miles in 16:00 min
Swim 1,350 yards in 45:00 min
Cycle 6 miles in 24:00 min

VI
Exercises Burning 250–299 Calories

Walk 4 miles in 1 hour 20:00 min
Walk/jog 2¼ miles in 27:00 min
Run 2½ miles in 20:00 min
Swim 2,400 yards in 1 hour 20:00 min
Cycle 12 miles in 1 hour 12:00 min

VII
Exercises Burning 300–349 Calories

Walk 5 miles in 1 hour 40:00 min
Walk/jog 2¾ miles in 39:00 min
Run 3 miles in 24:00 min
Swim 1,350 yards in 24:00 min
Cycle 9 miles in 24:00 min

VIII
Exercises Burning 350–399 Calories

Walk 5½ miles in 1 hour, 36:00 min
Walk/jog 3 miles in 36:00 min
Run 3½ miles in 28:00 min
Swim 1,350 yards in 36:00 min
Cycle 9 miles in 36:00 min

IX
Exercises Burning 400–449 Calories

Walk 6 miles in 1 hour 45:00 min
Walk/jog 3¾ miles in 45:00 min
Run 3¾ miles in 30:00 min
Swim 1,575 yards in 42:00 min
Cycle 10½ miles in 42:00 min

X
Exercises Burning 450–500 Calories

Walk 7 miles in 2 hours 20:00 min
Walk/jog 4 miles in 48:00 min
Run 4 miles in 32:00 min
Swim 1,800 yards in 48:00 min
Cycle 12 miles in 48:00 min